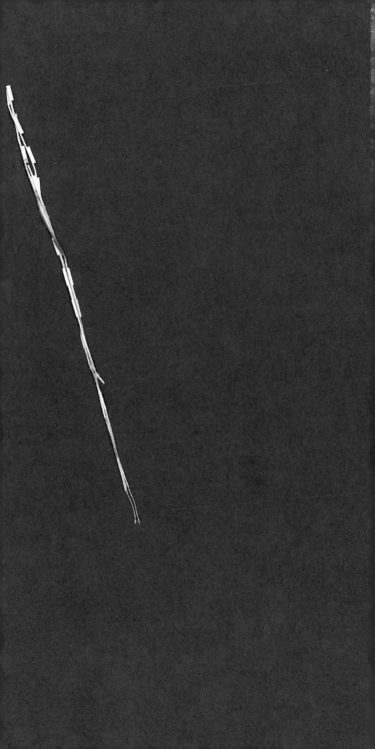

*The Nigel Lawson Diet Book*

*Also by Nigel Lawson*
The View from No. 11

# THE NIGEL LAWSON DIET BOOK

*Illustrated by Reginald Bass*

MICHAEL JOSEPH
London

MICHAEL JOSEPH LTD

Published by the Penguin Group

27 Wrights Lane, London w8 5tz
Viking Penguin Inc., 375 Hudson Street, New York, New York 10014, USA
Penguin Books Australia Ltd, Ringwood, Victoria, Australia
Penguin Books Canada Ltd, 10 Alcorn Avenue, Toronto, Ontario, Canada m4v 3b2
Penguin Books (NZ) Ltd, 182 – 190 Wairau Road, Auckland 10, New Zealand

Penguin Books Ltd, Registered Offices: Harmondsworth, Middlesex, England

First published 1996
1 3 5 7 9 10 8 6 4 2

Typeset in 12/15.5pt Monotype Perpetua
Typeset by Cambridge Phototypesetting Services
Printed and bound in Great Britain by
Clays Ltd, St Ives plc

A CIP catalogue record for this book is available from the British Library
ISBN 0 7181 4175 X

To Thérèse

*Without whom this book manifestly
could not have been written*

# Contents

———

PART ONE

*His Story*

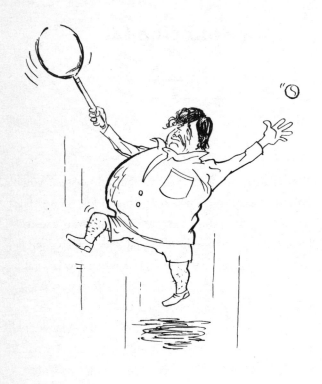

# On Being Fat

———

You already want to lose weight, otherwise you would scarcely be reading this book. That is important; for while extremes of all kinds are to be avoided, it is no sin to be fat – or overweight, to use the term that I preferred when I was a fat man. The last thing I wish to do is to try to persuade anyone to lose weight, nor would it serve any useful purpose. But if you have, for whatever reason, already firmly decided that that is what you wish to do, then this book may be of some help.

Looking back, I cannot remember when I first became fat: it was an insidiously gradual process. Although never skinny, I was certainly not a fat schoolboy, nor was I fat at Oxford or during my time in the Navy. It started to creep up on me some time after I had become a journalist, and particularly after I had passed my thirty-fifth birthday.

It was about that time that my elder son, Dominic, recalls that he and his sisters started to tease me about my increasing girth – usually at family meal times, when I was tucking in with some gusto – and to urge me to lose weight. To which I would reply that dieting would be 'my retirement job – a state I have yet to attain. I think at the time I meant it; although, had they challenged me a decade or so later, I might have borrowed Margaret Thatcher's mantra about sterling's entry into the European Monetary System's exchange rate mechanism, and told them, with rather greater accuracy, that I would do it when the time was right.

Certainly, I did not believe the time to be right then. I had always enjoyed eating and drinking, and always had a healthy appetite. Maybe this had something to do with having been a child during the war, when food was severely rationed. It was this experience, I suspect, which gave me the compulsion, which remained with me until I embarked on my diet half a century later, and which I have now mastered only with some difficulty, to finish everything on my plate, leaving nothing. Indeed, I frequently used to finish off what the children had left on their plates as well. It was the war,

too, which may have subconsciously led me to
view eating well as something to be savoured not
merely for its own sake but as the prize of peace
and victory.

## JOURNALIST'S TRADE

Be that as it may, what is clear is that lunching is
an integral part of the journalist's trade. It is over
the lunch table that he develops his relationships
with his sources of information, and indeed
garners much of that information; and the better
the journalist does in his career the better the
lunches tend to become. (The converse, however,
cannot be relied upon, whatever some journalists
may like to think.)

I suppose it was when, in 1960, I became the
principal author of the 'Lex' column of the *Financial
Times* – which at that time enjoyed a virtual
monopoly of critical comment on corporate affairs
– that I was first introduced to the pleasures of
the boardroom, and in particular the City boardroom, lunch. And when, the following year, I left
the *FT* to become the first City Editor of the
brand-new *Sunday Telegraph*, these lunching oppor-
tunities inevitably multiplied and, freed from the
daily treadmill, I had more time to devote to them.

This was perhaps just as well. In those long-gone days the City lunch was traditionally a heavy and leisurely affair; and the first time I lunched at Rothschilds, then still in their lovely old building in New Court, with its comfortable Edwardian country-house atmosphere, their unique and eccentric practice of rising from the table shortly after two o'clock came as something of a shock. Subsequently, as Editor of *The Spectator*, I exchanged the City and boardroom lunches for equally protracted meals with Ministers and senior civil servants at some of the best restaurants in London – all, needless to say, still in the stern cause of professional duty.

When, while still at *The Spectator*, I fought my first (and, happily, my only unsuccessful) general election campaign (at Slough, in 1970) I was assured by all the old political hands that I was bound to take off some weight. Every candidate, I was told, loses weight during the stress and strain, the hustle and bustle, the rushed and missed meals of campaigning in a marginal constituency. Not so: I did not lose so much as an ounce.

## POLITICAL LIFE

So by the time I had found a safe seat and finally left journalism for politics, when I had turned forty, the upward trend of my weight was already firmly established. To adapt the bard, sweet are the causes of obesity. I had by then made one or two attempts at dieting, but they did not last long and had little immediate and certainly no lasting effect. I had switched from taking sugar to taking saccharine with my coffee: a futile gesture if ever there was one. I had even gone to the length of spending a week in 1971 at a ludicrously expensive health farm, where I consumed nothing but water with a slice of lemon in it, as a result of which I felt so weak that I could do little more than sit feebly in front of a television set (and even then I could only watch BBC, as ITV appeared to carry nothing but food advertisements, which I found unbearable). Whatever I lost that week I put back on within days of returning to civilization.

Political life, perhaps inevitably for someone who was by now a fully paid-up member of the obese tendency, served only to accentuate the trend. If eating and drinking in the course of duty is an inescapable part of the journalist's trade, it is an even more integral part of political, and in particular ministerial, life. To the professional lunch was added the professional dinner, and much else besides. And as a Minister, which I was from the outset of the first Thatcher Government in 1979, the omnipresent official car and driver ensured that I never had to walk anywhere – not that it would have made any difference if I had. To be sure, the quality of the food and drink on offer was seldom particularly distinguished; but it was there, and it was consumed. It was also, of course, usually free; so there was not even the constraint of a bill to be paid at the end of the day.

But as every economically literate person knows, there is no such thing as a free lunch; and the politician frequently has to sing for his supper by making a post-prandial speech. This can in some cases inhibit the appetite. The most extreme instance I know was Harold Macmillan, who felt physically sick before any important speech, and simply could not eat a thing. This became so much a way of life that I remember sitting next to him, at a rather good private dinner he was to address well into his premiership, and watching him sit with an empty plate in front of him as he resolutely refused everything he was offered.

Alas, I am at the other end of the spectrum, and find it hard to speak, or function effectively in almost any way for that matter, on an empty stomach. As a result, I developed the bad habit, which to this day I have not been able to break, of eating fast, so as to give me time to compose myself and focus on what I am going to say in the interval between finishing my meal and standing up to speak.

## WEIGHT-WATCHERS

For some time I had become increasingly self-conscious and uneasy about my weight, or rather my girth. But it still came as something of a shock, when I became sufficiently well known as a Minister to be the subject of political cartoons, to discover that my most obvious physical characteristic, apart from my hair, of which I had plenty, was my pronounced fatness. Moreover, my self-consciousness at this discovery was intensified by the fact that, as Financial Secretary to the Treasury during the worst days of the recession of the early 1980s, it was part of my job to travel the country making speeches about how British industry was becoming leaner and fitter. Thankfully, and indeed importantly, *it* was; but *I* most certainly was not.

Even so, I still did nothing about it. It was not as if my obesity made me noticeably unwell. I am fortunate enough to have been born with a particularly robust constitution (the most important attribute, after luck, for a successful political career: far more important than, for example, intelligence) and have suffered scarcely a day's illness throughout my life. And I enjoy good food and wines. But the main reason for my inertia was that I thought that doing anything about it at that time would be too difficult and too doubtful of success.

There was the fact of my, admittedly few, previous attempts at slimming, to no avail, in the past. The most farcical of these occurred shortly after I had become a Minister, when my *bon vivant* parliamentary colleague, Spencer le Marchant, persuaded me to join his House of Commons weight-watchers club. Spencer was a huge mountain of a man, who fittingly represented a constituency by the name of High Peak, and whom I had come to know quite well during my brief sojourn in the Tory whips' office in Opposition in the mid-1970s.

His great contribution to the Conservative cause, during his seven years as a whip, most of it in Opposition, was to ensure that those of his colleagues who were fighting contentious legislation, line by line, upstairs in Committee through the watches of the night, were properly victualled. He carried out this self-appointed role, whenever requested, in considerable style, and I was frequently a beneficiary. As Napoleon had long ago observed, these things matter in battle.

Spencer's weight-watchers club, an annual event, began with a convivial champagne party to which MPs of all parties were invited; all members paid their £5 subscription and were weighed in and their weights duly recorded. A month later there was to be another champagne party, when all would be weighed again; and whoever had lost most weight over the intervening period was declared the winner and would collect all the £5 subscriptions. For a week after the initial event I made a point of eating rather less than usual, and then forgot about it. When the time came for the second weigh-in, to my embarrassment, I had actually put on a couple of pounds. The winner, I seem to recall, was Spencer himself.

There was no doubt, or so I told myself, that as a Minister the nature of the political life was not conducive to dieting. It was a matter not only of the lunches and the dinners, the receptions and even the banquets, with which it was studded, but also, at least after I had become Chancellor in 1983, of the relentless and all-consuming pressure of the job, which made me disinclined to devote even a small corner of my mind to focusing on matters of diet. Not that ministerial eating is all a matter of staggering from one official lunch, dinner, reception or banquet to the next: far from it. When the pressure is on, you are just as likely to snatch a quick sandwich lunch at your desk. But then your mind is even less on what you are eating.

## GASTRONOMIC DELIGHTS

There were some genuine gastronomic highlights, but they were few and far between. Not surprisingly, the French did things best: they have, after all, a reputation and a tradition to maintain, and it is expected of them. Moreover, while the average standard of eating out in France has declined, whereas ours has risen, over the past half century, their best remains superb.

The greatest *tour de force* I recall occurred towards the end of my time in office, when France held the rotating presidency of what was then still called the European Community, and its Socialist Government invited all the Finance Ministers and Central Bank Governors of the member countries to a weekend at one of the great luxury hotels of the world, the Hotel du Cap/Eden Roc at Cap d'Antibes, on the Riviera. Our suite, one of the best in the hotel, was priced at £2,000 a night. I shall always be grateful to the French taxpayer for footing the bill for an experience I would otherwise never have been able to afford. My wife,

Thérèse, who in general didn't much care for official travelling, sensibly chose to accompany me on that occasion, and we both recall in particular an exquisite mesclun which opened my eyes, for the first time in my life, to the potential of salad.

The home team's official entertaining, whether at the Mansion House, Number 10, Chequers, Buckingham Palace or Windsor Castle, was never quite up to the best French standards so far as the food was concerned, although the service could be, and on royal occasions invariably was, impeccable. Where we could, and occasionally did, score on non-royal occasions was in the wine department, for the Government Hospitality Service possesses a very fine cellar indeed. When the charming, intelligent and dignified Edouard Balladur became Finance Minister of France in 1986 I decided to invite him over to London for a tête-à-tête, or what is known in Whitehall jargon as a bilateral. Our talks were punctuated by a small luncheon at 11 Downing Street, the Chancellor's official residence, at which I was able to offer him a claret whose magnificence quite bowled him over.

Next door, while Margaret Thatcher's insistence on serving English, rather than French, mineral water was thoroughly commendable, I did feel that her tendency from time to time to ignore the glories of the GHS cellar and serve English

wine was perhaps taking patriotism a trifle too far.
But she was at all times intensely and admirably
practical; and never more so than in her brilliant
trick, as she sat down to the dinner table, of
deftly and unobtrusively hitching up any parts of
her attire, within decency, that might otherwise
have got unnecessarily creased.

However, if we could not quite compete with
the French on the food front, we were streets ahead
of the Americans. Perhaps it is enough to say that
the best official meals they provided were the
working breakfasts I had from time to time with
the US Treasury Secretary of the day – first, the
rough diamond Don Regan, and subsequently the
smoothly polished Jim Baker. Where I really did
eat well in Washington was when staying, which
I did once or twice a year as Chancellor, at Edwin
Lutyens' imposing British Embassy residence, where
the chefs were British, too. It is, in my experience,
the best hotel on the diplomatic circuit, with our
splendid eighteenth-century Paris Embassy, tucked
away behind its massive security gates in the chic
rue du Faubourg St Honoré, a close second.

But the most annoying feature of official lunches
and dinners in Washington was the American
habit of failing to provide a menu to let you know
what you were eating and drinking, something
unheard of in either Britain or France, or any-

where else in Europe so far as I can recall. It was, I suppose, a sign that they didn't really care. This failure was equally evident at the international organizations based in Washington. Even at the IMF, two successive French managing directors failed to remedy this defect; and the food and drink were correspondingly undistinguished.

I suspect I dined pretty well during the Tokyo Summit of 1986, but at that time I had not yet acquired a taste for Japanese food (which I now have). The most memorable occasion there, for me at any rate, was not the final banquet at the Imperial Palace, where the ancient Japanese music played throughout the meal on authentic period instruments was something for which, unlike the food, I shall never acquire a taste, but the dinner given to the G7 Finance Ministers the previous night at the Restaurant Kitcho by the then Finance Minister, the sage and wily Noboru Takeshita, where we were well looked after by a group of highly trained geisha girls. In that cultural setting it was just as well that none of the G7 countries had a female finance minister.

One practical footnote, as it were, for any man going for the first time to a traditional formal dinner in Japan, whether or not there are geishas present: make sure your socks are immaculate, as you will be dining with your shoes off.

## PRESSURES OF WORK

Looking back, it was not the quality of the food and drink on offer at official entertainments that persuaded me to consume more than I should have done. It was more the fact that, when one goes to occasions not because one wants to, but because one is obliged to, one is inclined to eat and, perhaps even more, to allow one's glass to be filled and to drink from it, out of boredom, or simply for something to do. But of course you can still say no. It is remarkable how large a part of the art of living, from filling (or not filling) one's engagement diary to bringing up young children, consists of the ability to say no and to stick to it; and how many people find the task beyond them. It is the same in government; notably, but by no means exclusively, in the case of the control of public spending.

When it comes to eating and drinking, it is probably harder (or so I told myself) when one is in a high-pressure job and one's mind is preoccupied with the problems that go with it. That was one excuse I had. Another was the long hours. As Chancellor I used to start work on weekdays at six in the morning, and aimed to stop by midnight. This gave me all the sleep I needed. But it is inevitably the case that the longer one is awake, the more time there is for eating and drinking. There were also more ministerial red boxes, typically at least a couple of them, filled with official submissions and papers of one kind or another, to be read over the weekend and fitted in around the usual Saturday constituency engagements; but this required neither particularly early starts nor late nights.

Since the objective of most of these constituency occasions was to raise funds for the Conservative cause locally, the much-maligned Tory ladies who habitually organized these functions understandably did not want to spend too much money on the food and drink, and it showed. But it would have been discourteous not to partake. The best bet, I found, was the straightforward wine and-cheese do – not because of the wine, which was probably what originally made me a confirmed whisky-drinker, but because, having the good fortune to represent a Leicestershire constituency, the cheeses I was able to choose from invariably included that king of the cheeseboard, Stilton.

It would have been perfectly possible to have been a rather more laid-back Chancellor and not worked those long hours during the week, as a number of occupants of that post have demonstrated. I chose not to be. This was not because I am a workaholic: I am far from that; and indeed when I held the now-defunct post of Secretary of State for Energy in the early 1980s, for example, my workload was substantially less time-consuming, and I had no desire to make it any greater than it had to be. Indeed, although active by temperament, I have to engage in a constant struggle against an innate laziness. But as Chancellor I was not content merely to keep the show on the road, important though that is, but sought also to engage in a thoroughgoing process of tax reform, privatization, deregulation, and various other reforms. And that inevitably took more time.

The most sensible way of reducing a Chancellor's workload, I believe, would be to move as I have long advocated to a genuinely independent, but accountable, Bank of England (although that is not why I favour it). It would be a distinct improvement over the present less than satisfactory halfway house.

## ALL IN THE GENES

But I digress. For the best excuse I had for being overweight, and doing nothing about it, was nothing to do with the demanding job I was doing or my hours of work. It was the consoling thought that my fatness was not my fault but rather an inescapable genetic inheritance of obesity: there was no running away from the fact that all four of my grandparents had been fat. Indeed one of them, my paternal grandfather, had died in his early seventies because the disease from which he suffered required an operation and the doctors had decided that he was too fat for a successful operation to be possible.

In fact, it is not entirely true that I did nothing about it. Within a year of becoming Chancellor, I fell into conversation with the incomparable and irreplaceable Willie Whitelaw, who told me that he had lost weight by giving up drinking spirits entirely and confining his alcoholic intake to wine. Despite my fondness for whisky, particularly malt whisky, I decided to do the same. Unfortunately, however, I did not lose any weight the Whitelaw way. I just drank more wine than before to replace the whisky. But at least I seemed to stop putting it on (by this time I weighed well over 16 stone, much too much for a man not quite 5 foot 9 inches tall) so I stuck to this regime.

But that is all I did; and over the next ten years, both in and out of office, I made no further attempts to lose weight. I simply consoled myself with the belief that at least I had at long last stabilized. Even this was an example of the sort of wishful thinking to which fatties are prone: what had really happened was that the upward trend had slowed sufficiently to enable me to wear the same suits until I felt that it was time for a new suit anyway.

Had I known, as I do now, how straightforward and relatively painless it would be to lose all the weight I wished to lose, despite my genetic pre-disposition, I would have done so a great deal sooner. It would probably have been slightly harder to diet successfully when I was Chancellor, if only because I might have found it harder to give the process the degree of attention it initially requires – but it would have been perfectly possible.

## WRITING MY MEMOIRS

Not that I embarked on a diet once I had resigned as Chancellor towards the end of 1989. Once I had weathered the difficult process of adjusting to the inevitably abrupt and in my case high-profile change from high office to normal life, which took some time, I embarked on the job of writing my

memoirs. Doing this, while remaining a Member
of Parliament and taking on a few business com-
mitments to make up for the money I had not
earned as a Minister, proved to be the hardest
task I had ever undertaken in my life. Few things
are more difficult than writing honestly and objec-
tively about one's own successes and failures in
the public arena, at a time when these continue
to be a matter of some controversy and lack of
objectivity on the part of others. Nor did I make
it any easier for myself by writing, in *The View
from No. 11*, a very long and, perhaps appropriately enough, given my shape at that time,
very fat book. During this exceptional phase, not
only did I make no attempt to focus my mind on
dieting, but I am pretty sure I was right not to
do so.

But I have no excuse whatever for doing
nothing about it after I had completed the book,
with an immense sense of relief and liberation,
in the summer of 1992. People used to ask me
whether I had enjoyed writing it. I would tell
them the truth: that I had hated writing it, but
enjoyed having written it.

## FITNESS MATTERS

As it was, it took a very specific event to persuade me to take the matter in hand. This was
the sudden emergence, while on a brief visit to
New York in the spring of 1994, of a pain in my
right knee sufficiently bad to make it impossible
to walk without a limp. Indeed, my mobility
was sufficiently impaired to make a nonsense of
playing tennis, by then virtually my only serious
form of exercise, as well as one of life's minor
pleasures. When, after a few days back in
England, this apparently transatlantic curse infuri-
atingly refused to go away, I went to see our
excellent local GP, Dewi Roberts, now, alas, re-
tired. I was dismayed to learn from him that I
was suffering from a mildly but uncomfortably
arthritic knee.

The immediate crisis was fairly readily dealt
with. A visit to the local hospital for an arthroscopy,
during which a specialist poked around inside
my knee (the wonders of keyhole surgery: into
hospital at breakfast time and out again by lunch-
time), coupled with anti-inflammatory painkiller
drugs to be taken whenever needed, ensured that
the pain and the limp went and my mobility and
tennis were substantially restored. But Dewi

helpfully pointed out that the arthritis, which was essentially simply the result of wear and tear of that most complicated of all joints, the knee, was hardly surprising given the enormous amount of weight my knees had had to bear, year in, year out; and that, if I did not reduce that weight, which by then, I was appalled to discover, had edged up further to only two pounds short of 17 stone, the condition would inevitably worsen.

It was this spectre of impaired mobility that tipped the balance. Whereas, hitherto, the joys of the table and general inertia had combined to overcome both the dictates of vanity and my wife's constant urging over many years to lose weight, this was something serious. Moreover, it had come little more than a year after an earlier embarrassing clash between my obesity and my previous sporting fitness. In my youth I had been a keen skier, and while my style was undistin guished I was fast enough to ski for the Oxford second six in the Varsity race. I continued with the sport, at first regularly and then intermittently until, having reached the age of forty and with none of my first family of children showing any great interest in it, I gave it up and took to occasional water-skiing instead.

Then, after a gap of more than twenty years,

the family decided to go to Davos in January 1993 to take part in the annual Parliamentary ski expedition. On only our second day there, and only his second day on skis ever, my younger son, Tom, had the great misfortune to suffer a nasty fall and break his shoulder badly, spending the rest of a blighted holiday in hospital, where he had to undergo a complicated operation. Since the main purpose of the exercise had been to initiate my two younger children into the joys of skiing, the holiday was clearly an unmitigated failure. But it was something of a personal failure for me, too.

In between hospital visits, telephone calls to the insurance company's doctor, and the various other consequences of poor Tom's accident, I was able to get some skiing in. It all came back to me, somewhat rustily, without too much difficulty, except for one major and wholly unexpected problem. I found that, because of my great weight, if I fell I was usually unable to get up again without calling on someone else to assist me: a thoroughly humiliating experience. This gave me a terror of falling which I had never felt before, and obliged me to ski in a ludicrously timid fashion which took most of the fun out of it.

I responded to that uncomfortable piece of self-knowledge by resolving to give up skiing for good, as young Tom had done in the light of his far worse experience. But the knee episode was altogether more serious. I decided that, for the first time in my life, I would go on an effective diet and stick to it.

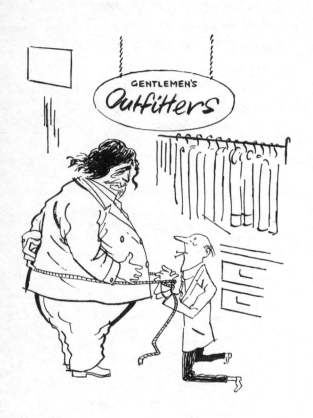

# 2

# On Becoming Thin

———

But what diet? As a lifelong fattie, I was already fairly well aware, albeit without ever having been sufficiently motivated to read a diet book, of the various sorts of diet that people talk about and occasionally put into practice. It is, after all, one of the more useful fall-back topics at difficult or dull dinner parties.

## CONSIDERING DIETS

It was easier to decide what not to do than what to do. I was clear from the outset that I did not want to have anything to do with pills or injections, whether to suppress the appetite or for any other dietary purpose. Being over-weight – and I am not of course referring here to extreme cases of obesity – is not to my mind an illness, and I had no wish to treat it as one.

Equally, I did not want to resort to patent slimming products of any kind. Rightly or wrongly, I have always been both sceptical of the claims made for these and repelled by the thought of consuming them. I wanted to continue to eat real food, particularly the kind of food I enjoy most.

One possible approach, at least in theory, would have been to give myself a sufficiently modest ration of calories for each day, and make sure that what I ate and drank during the day was always within the prescribed limits. This can work in practice, too: my good friend Tony Jay, co-author of that most perceptive of all studies of British government in practice, the TV series *Yes, Minister* and *Yes, Prime Minister*, had lost four stone that way, more than twenty years previously, and succeeded in keeping it off.

First, he studied the calorie charts and switched from high to low-calorie food and drink. Then, with the aid of a pocket chart which he always carried with him, he carefully calculated the calorie count of absolutely everything he consumed and, by this system of what he described as 'zero-based calorie accounting', ensured that his daily calorie intake was always significantly lower than his calorie output.

This accountancy approach worked for him, but I was sure it would not work for me. Counting the calories of everything that passed down my gullet was much too complicated, much too time-consuming, and much too boring for me, perhaps because of the innate laziness to which I have already confessed. I knew that I simply would not have been able to keep it up. He did, because this meticulous approach clearly appealed to his particular cast of mind, and the ingenuity expended in balancing the calories consumed against the satisfaction derived, and mastering the calorific–felicific calculus required, gave him sufficient intellectual satisfaction to persist.

## THE MOTIVATIONAL FACTOR

We have, however, now come to the heart of the matter. *The secret of successful dieting lies in psychology.* All dieting is a matter of self-discipline. The trick is to find an approach that makes the maintenance of the necessary self-discipline as easy as possible. And that, to repeat, is a matter of personal psychology. At the beginning *there has to be a sufficiently strong motivational trigger*. For me it was the knee problem; for others it will doubtless be something else. Most doctors understandably home in on the well-known health risks associated with obesity. Certainly, if you start looking out for really old fat people, you will find there are not many of them, and in particular, very few really old fat men. Living to a ripe old age may well be an overrated pastime, but the doctors have a point. At any rate, the non-obese pay lower life assurance premiums.

The motivational trigger, however, while necessary, is only the start. The nature of the diet itself has to be one that makes the self-discipline required to stick to it as easy as possible. What I now describe is a method which, in those terms, undoubtedly worked for me. In less than a year I lost five stone, going from just under 17 stone to just under 12 stone, without too much difficulty; and I have maintained my new weight ever since. In terms of weight, some 30 per cent of me has, relatively painlessly, disappeared.

Looking at it another way, during the period in which I was losing weight, I lost it, on average, at the rate of about a pound and a half a week. Losing a pound and a half may seem, at first sight, a trifling matter. What makes it significant is how it clocks up over time. It implies losing very nearly half a stone a month; so that, after six months, which is not a long time in anyone's life, you will (if you continue with the diet) be the best part of three stone lighter.

My actual progress was not, of course, linear: not surprisingly, the easiest stone to lose was the first. During the first month of my diet, I found I was losing some three pounds a week; and the weekly rate of loss gradually diminished as time went by. But the point is not to be discouraged by the apparent modesty of your initial weight loss. After all, when you were putting on weight, it was in all probability a far more gradual process even than this, yet the cumulative effect was all too perceptible.

The diet method I used may well not work for everyone, although I would be astonished if it didn't benefit most people. I adopted it only after one or two false starts. Initially, I went to see a Harley Street doctor who had been recommended to me as an expert on dieting. His patent regime may well have worked, but it was so extreme and unbalanced in the shortlist of foods it permitted that it had to be supplemented by pills to prevent constipation and regular vitamin injections to make good the deficiency in the diet itself. That was not the sort of thing that appealed to me at all. When I told Dewi, our local doctor, about it, he dismissed it as a load of nonsense, and gave me instead the standard, medically approved diet sheet to read. This was no doubt full of common sense, but, like the pudding which Winston Churchill famously rejected at the Savoy Hotel, it lacked a theme. So I decided to devise a method of my own, one that made sense in psychological as well as dietary terms.

<br>

## KEY PRINCIPLES

**The guiding principle is to keep it simple.**

I first decided on a target for the amount of weight I wanted to lose. Like any other target, this had to be ambitious enough to be worth going for, but not so ambitious as to seem unrealistic. In my case I plumped for roughly three stone, which implied a target weight of, say, $13\frac{1}{2}$ stone.

I was well aware that, even if I achieved this, I would still be overweight. My body mass index, or BMI, calculated (thus does metrication sweep all before it) by dividing one's weight in kilos by the square of one's height in metres, which at its peak stood at 35, would still have come down only to 28. And according to the Royal Society of Medicine's *Encyclopaedia of Family Health*, anyone, male or female, with a BMI greater than 27 – a condition, it says, that applies to some one-fifth of British men and a quarter of British women – can consider themselves to be obese. But $13\frac{1}{2}$ stone still seemed a good enough target to be getting on with: I had known a number (albeit a rather small number) of fat men who had lost three stone, and seen the difference it made to them.

In parenthesis, and for the benefit of those who wish to check their BMI and don't want to go to the trouble of converting their weight into kilos (one stone = 6.35 kilos) or their height into metres (one foot = 0.305 metres) I have provided a simple ready reckoner. If your BMI is above the stepped box, you are, in the eyes of the medical profession, incontrovertibly obese. If your BMI is within the stepped box, there is no obvious medical reason for you to bother about your weight. If your BMI is below the stepped box, you are underweight, and should not be reading this book.

Somewhat surprisingly, given the marked difference in build between the two sexes, neither the Royal Society of Medicine's encyclopaedia nor what little other recent literature I have seen draws a distinction between men and women so far as BMI acceptability is concerned. Do my nostrils detect just the faintest whiff of political correctness in this unisex approach? Certainly, inasmuch as the BMI is a useful guide, I suspect that men would do best to aim for the upper half of the stepped box, while women would feel happier in the lower half.

## BMI READY RECKONER

|  |  | *Height in feet and inches* | | | | | |
|---|---|---|---|---|---|---|---|
|  |  | 5' | 5'3" | 5'6" | 5'9" | 6' | 6'3" |
| *Weight in stones* | 18 | 49 | 44 | 41 | 37 | 34 | 31 |
|  | 17 | 46 | 42 | 39 | 35 | 32 | 29 |
|  | 16 | 43 | 40 | 36 | 33 | 30 | 27 |
|  | 15 | 41 | 37 | 34 | 31 | 28 | 26 |
|  | 14 | 38 | 35 | 32 | 29 | 26 | 24 |
|  | 13 | 35 | 32 | 30 | 27 | 24 | 22 |
|  | 12 | 33 | 30 | 27 | 25 | 22 | 21 |
|  | 11 | 30 | 27 | 25 | 23 | 21 | 19 |
|  | 10 | 27 | 25 | 23 | 21 | 19 | 17 |
|  | 9 | 24 | 22 | 21 | 19 | 17 | 15 |
|  | 8 | 22 | 20 | 18 | 17 | 15 | 14 |
|  | 7 | 19 | 17 | 16 | 15 | 13 | 12 |

The other dimension to targets is, of course, the time allowed to achieve them. As with the process of economic or indeed any other reform, progress has to be fast enough to be perceptible and create confidence that there is light at the end of the tunnel and that the inconveniences of adjustment are worthwhile, but not so fast as to precipitate crisis and unsustainability. It was on this principle, for example, that Geoffrey Howe and I settled on the annual numbers for monetary growth and the budget deficit in the original Medium-Term Financial Strategy in 1980. I was not at all sure how long I should allow myself to reach my target weight, but it clearly needed to be a matter of months rather than years — and months rather than weeks, too, although I was determined that I would see results after the first month.

In all aspects of life, a sense of achievement powerfully helps to keep one going. I adopted the rule of weighing myself regularly each weekend. The fact that each reading was slightly but perceptibly less than the previous one not only gave me that sense of achievement which crucially reinforced the self-discipline that lies at the heart of any successful diet. It also meant that, by dividing my target loss of weight by the average weekly weight loss I seemed to be securing, I could give myself a rough idea of when that target might be attained.

In the event, I found I had lost almost a stone by the end of the first month, and reached my target weight after six months or so. By then the regime had proved to be so successful – I had not only lost all the weight I had originally set out to lose, but felt decidedly better, too – that I continued for a further three months or so, during which time I shed another stone to get down to $12\frac{1}{2}$ stone. This seemed a good time to ease up and switch to a more relaxed diet, so as to stabilize my weight at its new and greatly reduced level.

I actually lost a further half stone and more, before finally stabilizing at just under 12 stone, implying a reassuringly healthy BMI of below 25. According to the Consumers' Association's *Fit and Healthy at 40+*, a somewhat painful publication which Thérèse, as a member of the Council of that organization, obliged me to read, a BMI in the 20 to 25 range is 'ideal' – although for myself, I would regard anything in the lower half of that range as far from ideal.

## THE REDUCING DIET

So, there are really two diets: the reducing diet until you have reached your target weight, and subsequently a maintenance diet to stay at or around your target weight. This may well, as in my case, be a revised target after the original one has been attained: there is nothing wrong in that – provided, of course, you don't take it too far.

What, then, of the reducing diet? The guiding principle, as I have said, is to keep it simple. This means, in the first place, sticking to a few simple rules.

The thinking behind this is that *what you are seeking to do is to change your eating habits*. It is almost as easy to fall into good habits as it is to fall into bad habits, if you put your mind to it. And once you have developed a habit, that is what, for the most part, you will actually *want* to do: the need for self-discipline and self-restraint becomes very much less. The Chinese *want* to eat Chinese food, the Japanese, Japanese food, the Italians, Italian food, and so on, because that is what they are in the habit of eating.

The easiest way to change your eating habits is thus to *adopt a small number of simple rules, and then stick to them over a sufficient period of time*. This approach clearly eliminates crash diets, which in any case are probably undesirable for a number of other reasons. But it also, for my money, rules out the calorie-counting system, which is far too complicated for a simple soul like me to become the second nature which a habit has to be.

The approach which I adopted may well not be the only way to diet successfully: I am sure it is not. But it is clearly the way best suited to the busy executive, who frequently has to have his or her meals on the job, and whose mind has to be focused firmly on the topic under discussion rather than the food on the plate. The adoption of a small number of simple rules, which rapidly become habits, makes dieting almost an automatic process, and frees the conscious mind for other purposes.

Of course, as you approach your final target weight you have, to some extent, to acquire yet another set of habits, as you switch from the reducing diet to the maintenance diet. But since the latter is essentially a modified and relaxed version of the former, this second change is unlikely to be a problem. Indeed, it feels like a treat. So it is the simple rules for the reducing diet that are effectively the key to success.

**The first of these rules, and for me the most difficult, and it was very difficult, was initially to cut out alcohol altogether.**

While I was losing weight, that is to say, for some nine months or so, I was on the wagon. There is no getting away from the dismal fact that all alcoholic drink is extremely fattening. Not only that, but if I take alcohol at meal times I tend to linger longer over the meal, and as a result eat more as well – partly, no doubt, because alcohol tends to loosen resolve. But the critical denial is the alcohol itself, and the key question is how to make this temporary deprivation tolerable.

I suppose I could have compromised by drinking, say, one or two glasses of wine a day. But it would have been just as hard, indeed almost certainly harder, to stick rigidly to that as to abstain altogether. This is not merely because of the insidious way in which one drink so easily leads to another, but also because, when you are out, once you have accepted a drink, no one believes you will not take another, which creates a pressure the dieter can do without.

There is a Murphy's Law of parties, which ensures that the probability of an empty glass being filled varies inversely with the guest's desire for a drink. So, if you want to cut down on alcohol it is best not to have a wine glass in your hand in the first place – or, if you are seated, best not to have any in front of you. Quietly ask the waiter or whoever is responsible for serving the wine to remove them. Moreover, the great thing about total abstinence is that it hastens the day when your target weight is reached, and thus the day when you can switch to the maintenance diet in which alcohol, as we shall see, features in an agreeable way.

Even so, I was not strong enough simply to leave a vacuum where the alcohol had been, or to confine myself to water. The yearning for a drink around midday and again around six o'clock in the evening was too great: at these points I could tell the time without consulting my watch. So I decided to replace an exceedingly fattening addictive stimulant by a non-fattening addictive stimulant: caffeine. Except during meal times (when I did stick to water, usually of the fizzy variety) whenever I felt like a drink I would have either a black coffee, without sugar, or an ice-cold Diet Cola drink.

In the past, I had never touched the latter, finding it distinctly unappealing to the palate. But it was amazing how soon it became addictive, in a perfectly controlled way; which is no doubt why this curious product has become the best-known symbol of American culture throughout the world. I normally alternated the two forms of caffeine, having a black coffee at or after breakfast, a Diet Cola before lunch, a black coffee after lunch, a Diet Cola before dinner, and a black coffee after dinner. And, invariably, I stuck to Diet Cola at drinks parties – or cursed the host or hostess who failed to provide it.

**The second simple rule, and second prohibition I adopted, was no eating between meals.**

None at all. In no circumstances. This automatically ruled out a whole range of nibbles, from nuts to canapés to chocolates. Moreover, since I do not count tea as a meal, it also ruled out cakes and biscuits – not to mention my favourite companion to tea, cucumber sandwiches.

It may be that this second rule was unnecessarily rigid, too: no doubt there are things like sticks of celery which are innocent of anything that makes one fat. But for me it was psychologically easier to get out of the habit of nibbling between meals and into the habit of having nothing at all between meals than it would have been to embark on a policy of carefully controlled nibbling. For one thing, it required much less thought; and the more that dieting could take the form of automatic responses, and the less conscious thought involved, the better.

**There is, besides, an attractive counterpart to the rule of no eating between meals; and that is always to eat three proper meals a day – breakfast, lunch and dinner – with a clear conscience.**

They cannot, of course, be just any old meals. I decided to cut out a whole range of fattening or potentially fattening foods, and stick to those less fattening foods I liked best, of which I would then eat as much as I felt like. I was greatly helped by the fact that Thérèse is a superb cook, and provided me with excellent meals which conformed to those guidelines. (The second part of this book sets out a number of the meals she devised.) This was particularly important in that it enabled me to look on my diet not, primarily, as an act of renunciation, but as an opportunity to focus on the wide range of delicious foods and meals I could still eat. For me, at any rate, this positive approach was a key aspect of the psychology of successful dieting.

For breakfast, the only meal I cook myself, I preferred to stick to the same formula every day: two poached eggs, with the poaching cups greased with a drop of olive oil instead of butter, on a single slice of unbuttered toast, washed down with a glass of grapefruit juice, preferably fresh. For lunch and dinner, apart from fresh fruit I avoided desserts of all kinds; and in general would never knowingly eat any of the following:

PROHIBITED

**Fat** of all kinds (and most oil)
**Dairy products** (milk, butter, cream, cheese etc)
**Butter-based sauces** (e.g. hollandaise)
**Sugar** in any shape or form
**Fried food** of any description

**Starchy foods** (such as bread, potatoes, pasta, rice, batter and pastry)

These few prohibitions aside, a number of which clearly overlap, I would eat as much as I felt like of anything else, while in general making a point of avoiding second helpings – and when in doubt, going without. Abstention from milk, incidentally, had the consequence of automatically ruling out breakfast cereals and porridge, too: it also meant that I switched to taking tea with lemon (or, for preference, China tea by itself; a much cleaner taste anyway) and drinking my coffee black at all times.

What I did eat, then, consisted essentially of the following:

RECOMMENDED

**Fish and any other seafood**, provided it was not fried

**Meat**, except for the fatty bits

**Poultry and game**, avoiding any fat or skin

**Eggs**, if not fried

**Fruit** (especially fresh citrus fruit)

**Salads** (with lemon juice or oil-free dressing)

**Green vegetables** – and indeed vegetables of any other colour provided they were not particularly starchy

I use the term 'knowingly' about the prohibitions because it was perfectly clear, particularly when eating out, that some of the forbidden ingredients would have been used in the cooking. I did not allow that to worry me in the slightest. What we are talking about here is a diet, not a religion.

What I continued to eat happily embraced most of the things I had most enjoyed eating all my life, plus the addition of one element, salads, which I had hitherto regarded with considerable distaste. I am still at best indifferent to the all-too-prevalent garish mixed salad: it is always a good rule to avoid having anything that is visually displeasing on your plate, anyway. But, to my surprise, I have become a complete convert to the more interesting forms of green salad. I also enjoy the occasional red salad: tomato, kidney beans and red onion. But, to repeat, never mixed; and green is best.

I was well aware that the diet I had devised did not sit entirely happily with the current conventional nutritional wisdom, particularly so far as the omission of most carbohydrates was concerned. This did not worry me in the slightest. Over the years I had observed how the conventional nutritional wisdom was very much a thing of fashion, constantly changing. The great thing about my diet was that it suited me, that there were no untoward side effects, and that it worked.

Like any diet, mine was obviously easiest to follow at home; and even when forbidden foods such as potatoes were usually on offer, if only for the benefit of the children, Thérèse would always see to it that there was enough that conformed to the guidelines as well. Similarly, when eating out at restaurants, I could always pick and choose what I ate. But I even found that when eating out at boardroom lunches or dinner parties I could quietly follow the guidelines to a reasonable degree of approximation, without ever causing any awkwardness. While you yourself may be keenly aware of what you are eating or not eating, others will seldom notice unless you are unwise enough to draw attention to it. At any boardroom lunch or dinner party there was always a part, and usually a large part, of the meal that was reasonably compatible with my diet, and I would simply eat that and abstain from the rest. There is no need to be a fanatic on such occasions.

The biggest practical problem when eating out was, I suppose, remembering to decline any dessert, however attractive it looked. This was not too difficult for me, since I have never had a particularly sweet tooth. A friend of mine, who has, found that it helped him if, on his way to lunch or dinner, he rehearsed in his head the line 'Just coffee for me, please' so that it would come out automatically, on cue, when the time came. Clearly this rehearsal technique can also be applied to other temptations when lunching or dining out – perhaps most obviously to the alcoholic drink on offer.


## WHEN TO START

I have described how, by clinging to a small number of simple rules, which gradually evolved into a habit, dieting became increasingly less difficult for me as time passed. It is obviously hardest and most painful during the first two or three weeks (it certainly was for me), which means that it is sensible to take the trouble to start your new regime when the circumstances are psychologically most favourable.

It was for that reason that I started my own diet, and in particular my complete abstention from alcohol when we were on holiday abroad during the summer of 1994. I had previously been drinking, on average, almost a bottle and a half of wine a day, without any adverse effects apart from obesity. While this may seem perverse, in that holidays are a time to let yourself go, they are or should be, above all, a time when you are under least stress and strain, least time pressure, expending least energy, and a time when you are most free to focus your mind on what you are eating and drinking. In other words, they are in fact far and away the easiest time to exercise the self-discipline involved in beginning a diet.

It helps considerably if, as I did, you take your holiday in a hot country, since heat always tends to reduce the appetite, and in one that is not noted for the distinction of its cuisine or the quality of its wines, so that the temptation to eat and drink is minimized and with it the degree of sacrifice required. The Caribbean is ideal in this context, but there are other places much nearer to home, in North Africa, for example, that would fit the bill almost as well.

## BACK HOME

Once back in England, I asked Thérèse to devise a diet and prepare meals for me that conformed to the rules I have already set out, and which would at the same time prevent me from feeling hungry or deprived of the pleasures of the table.

She rose to the challenge magnificently. She knew me well enough to realize that preventing me from feeling hungry was as much a matter of providing meals on time as of the amount of food I ate. Over the years, my system had become accustomed to a regular routine: breakfast at eight, a drink at noon, lunch at one, a drink at six, and dinner at eight; and I would feel seriously hungry or alcohol-deprived, as the case may be, and become edgy and distracted, when one of these daily events was significantly delayed. (A cup of tea at half-past four could be forgone without serious withdrawal symptoms; and I had already abandoned my previous regular malt whisky nightcap when I largely gave up spirits in 1984.)

Thérèse realized that, such is the force of habit, punctuality could take much of the pain out of dieting. I found that one of the golden rules of dieting was not only not to eat at all between meals, when I didn't really feel hungry, merely tempted, but to eat reasonably promptly at the meal times to which I had become accustomed, when I did indeed feel hungry. On the rare occasions when I actually felt hungry between meals, the feeling soon passed — with the help, if need be, of a glass of fizzy water.

As for preventing me from being deprived of the pleasures of the table, this meant, first and foremost, adapting her style of cooking by finding less-fattening substitutes for many of the ingredients she had formerly used. In general, while the range of food I now eat is slightly narrower than it used to be, and the quantity slightly smaller, the quality, and thus the enjoyment, has not diminished at all: indeed, if anything, it has been enhanced. If this seems too good to be true, I would direct you to the sample meals included in the second part of this book.

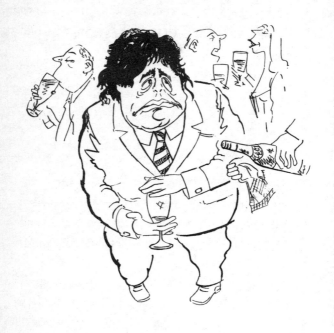

# 3

# On Staying Thin

___

So much for the *reducing* diet. What of the *maintenance* diet – the one I now live with? As I have already mentioned, it is essentially a modified and relaxed form of the reducing diet; but the modifications are significant.

The biggest difference is on the *drink* front. I continue to keep off spirits – except on the rare but cherished occasions when I am eating caviar, when vodka is an essential accompaniment – and beer, too, for that matter, but have gone back to drinking wine, in a controlled way. This control takes two forms. In the first place, except on special occasions, I normally stick to mineral water at lunch. Then, with dinner, I operate a quality threshold, drinking as much good wine as I feel like (usually red, whereas I used to be more of a white wine drinker), but no plonk at all. Dinner at home is normally washed down with a decent, if unspectacular, 1990 claret. I find that this simple rule greatly enhances the quality of life, and can be adhered to without any embarrassment. When I find myself at a dinner where an indifferent wine is being offered, I politely decline on the grounds that I am driving.

So far as *eating* is concerned, I have removed from the prohibited list cheese, plus oatcakes when eating the cheese, and (non-fried) rice, chiefly so that I can enjoy the occasional Chinese or Indian meal, or one of Thérèse's delicious Italian-style risottos. I no longer bother to remove the skin when eating poultry. I also allow myself to eat pasta once a week, and my favourite dessert, summer pudding – but no others. And, of course, blinis and sour cream with the caviar. One great advantage of being chairman of a company that specializes in doing business in Central and Eastern Europe is that I have a ready source of reasonably priced caviar.

This, however, is simply the way I have chosen to relax my own diet. Others may well choose to do it differently. For example, I could just as well have restored potatoes, if cooked in a non-fatty way, rather than pasta and rice, to my regular diet. The reward for reaching your final target weight is that you can then relax your regime to include, within quantitative reason, whatever hitherto forbidden foods you missed most when you were reducing.

Even on my relaxed maintenance diet, it would be dishonest not to admit that there are some things that I still miss from time to time. Roast potatoes, shepherd's pie, steak and kidney pie, real mayonnaise, hollandaise sauce, Welsh rabbit, pork sausages, treacle tart, chocolate pots and malt whisky come to mind. I don't miss them much, however, for the simple reason that I so enjoy what I *do* eat. But if I were ever to feel a craving for any of these, I would indulge it – not, of course, as a matter of habit, but as a treat.

One of the golden rules of ministerial life is never say never: the future is far too uncertain. I remember how that nice man Henry Hopkinson, a junior colonial office minister in the 1950s, achieved a degree of fame he was unlikely to have achieved in the normal course of events, and sacrificed his future political career, by breaking this golden rule and assuring the House of Commons that the then British colony of Cyprus would never be given its independence.

In a happier sense, the dieter, too, should *never say never*. Losing weight (and, of course, keeping it off: there is little point in making the effort to lose weight if you are going to allow yourself to put it on again) need not mean that there is anything that you will *never* eat or drink again. For the few months that you are actually reducing, you will do best to be strict with yourself. During that phase, backsliding should be avoided: it undermines the habit-forming process you are engaged in and thus makes subsequent dieting much harder than it need be. But once you have reached your ultimate target weight, not only do you, necessarily, switch over to a much less stringent maintenance diet, but you have earned the reward of treating yourself to anything you like from time to time. Save your backsliding for then – and enjoy it. In essence, this is another aspect of the positive approach which, as I have already noted, is an important aspect of the psychology of successful dieting.

Some people, it must be said, are stricter than this. I have a high regard for the trim-figured Mervyn King, currently the Economics Director of the Bank of England. He was formerly one of the group of independent economists I used to consult from time to time during the last three years of my time as Chancellor, and I tried hard to persuade him to become my full-time Deputy Chief Economic Adviser. For many years he has been a rigorous and successful dieter and, so far as I am aware, will *never*, for example, allow himself both starch and protein in the same meal (a principle, I gather, of more than one well-known diet). He holds that, just as fighting inflation has to be an immutable way of life, with no let-up ever, so, too, does non-fattening eating. I believe he is right about inflation, but not about eating, where my own experience demonstrates that, once the reducing phase is over, this degree of rigidity is happily not required.

All this has been about food and drink, with not a word about *exercise*. The truth is that, while regular (but not excessive) exercise is no doubt terribly good for you, it is quite unnecessary if your object is simply to lose weight. Physical activity of the right kind, and indeed of most kinds, will help to keep you fit; but it would require a phenomenal amount of exercise to enable you to lose even a small amount of weight. For all practical purposes, if you want to lose weight, there is no substitute for dieting; and dieting is perfectly capable of doing the job on its own. That said, I do play more tennis than I used to, and play more freely with less weight to carry, and also from time to time make a point of walking up and down stairs, rather than taking the lift. But that is virtually all I do by way of exercise.

No doubt I ought to do more than that; but not a lot more, I suspect. For while one's body seems able to adjust without difficulty to quite a radical change of diet, exercise can be a much more violent and dangerous activity. When I was Chancellor, my most sporting and fitness-conscious junior minister was regularly afflicted by aches and pains of one kind or another, sometimes quite badly, from which I was entirely spared. I note, too, that, according to the press, Ms Jane Fonda, the high priestess of the work-out and aerobics religion, has recently (after making a small fortune from her preaching) given it up, claiming to have discovered that it was all a mistake.

Even so, I have little doubt that, from the point of view of fitness, the wisest course is to adopt a moderately rigorous exercise regime when young, and then stick to it throughout the rest of one's active life. But for those of us who omitted to take that course early on, to take up such a regime in later life would be asking for trouble. Moreover, it is as foolish to take any exercise that you don't enjoy as it would be to eat food that you don't enjoy. And, fortunately, exercise is wholly unnecessary if your sole object is to lose weight and reduce girth – although it may have some bearing on aspects of your body shape, if that is what turns you (and others) on.

What is all-important in this context is your diet, which is why it is more effective to let the animals and birds you eat do the exercise for you, so that they stay lean and healthy. Thus game, both feathered and furred, is ideal for the meat component of your diet. But, of course, the key to successful dieting is not so much the diet itself as your ability to stick to it. The essence of dieting is pretty obvious, when all is said and done: it is basically a matter of eating and drinking less in general, and of the more fattening things in particular. The difficult part is to have the self-discipline to stick to it.

**An important part of the solution to this lies in devising meals which, while conforming to the diet, are a pleasure to eat.**

It was here that Thérèse made her invaluable contribution.

### SIDE EFFECTS

That is not to say there are no drawbacks. The principal one is financial. As you lose weight, your clothes inevitably become too large for you. In my case, I lost twelve inches around the waist, going from 46 inches to 34 inches, and two inches around the neck, going from an 18-inch to a 16-inch collar size. So there is nothing for it but to buy a whole new set of clothes.

This is greatly complicated by the fact that you are unlikely to be sure at what size you will ultimately stabilize. The last thing you will want to do is to buy yourself a whole new wardrobe as soon as your existing clothes have become too big for you, only to lose still more girth and have to go through the process all over again.

On the other hand, few misfits are more obvious than a collar that is manifestly too large. So, unless you have a lifestyle in which you can dispense with wearing a tie and live permanently in open-neck shirts, turtle-neck sweaters and the like, you will be obliged to buy a small number of inexpensive new shirts to see you through the interim stage of the slimming process, while postponing all major sartorial investment until you are confident your size has stabilized.

Unlike shirts, other items of clothing – trousers, suits and even overcoats – can, of course, be taken in, and do not strictly need to be replaced. This clearly saves money, even though you are unlikely to look as good or feel as good as in clothes that really are the right size for you. Certainly, it would be foolish to buy any new clothes other than shirts until you have unquestionably settled down in your new weight and size. But to cope with the transitional stage you will probably need to have at least one of your suits altered at some point along

the way. The mistake I made was to have too many
suits and pairs of trousers altered prematurely.

If you are, as I was, seriously overweight, and
are thus seeking to lose, and do lose, a significant
amount of weight, it is not only your clothes that
will become too large for you: your skin may well
do, too. This will be particularly obvious at the
front of the neck and under the chin. Over time,
this surplus will to some extent adjust of its own
accord; but the older you are, the less likely it
is that the expansion of your skin that occurred
during your overweight years will be completely
reversed. You then have the choice of either
living with the resulting creases or patronizing that
branch of the surgical profession that specializes
in making the necessary alterations.

So far, rightly or wrongly, I have opted for the
former. It all depends, I suppose, on how much
your looks – as opposed to your health, fitness,
and general sense of well-being – matter to you;
and in my case my innate conservatism has played
a part. Yet I have to admit to a slight inconsis-
tency in taking the trouble of, and indeed some
pleasure in, buying new suits that fit me, while
not bothering to have my skin altered to fit me.

Whatever you decide to do on this front, be
warned that, although you will be widely com-
plimented on your achievement, most of your

friends will initially be distinctly disconcerted by your new slim appearance. Even I was slightly put out, at first, to discover the re-emergence of a ribcage which had been hidden for so many years that I had forgotten it existed. Other people, too, are innately conservative, and it will take time for them to come to terms with the fact that the physical reality no longer conforms to the mental image they have long had of you. Some people, indeed, may even fail to recognize you at first (as someone who has suffered from a surfeit of visual recognition, I found this no bad thing). Others will assume that you must be ill; while still others will tell you they preferred you as you were, either because they genuinely did, or because they are fat themselves, envious and wish to undermine you.

These last, however galling their observations may be, will be a minority; but if this sort of thing does worry you, the simple answer is to confine your weight loss to, say, three stone rather than the five stone which I ultimately decided to shed. Moreover, if you do decide to lose weight, remember that you are not doing it for others, you are doing it for yourself. This is one very good reason why, when you have done it, you should reward yourself by buying a completely new set of clothes which fit the new you, and which you will feel good in.

That, of course, presupposes that you are determined to stay slim.

**Clearly, the ultimate test of a successful approach to dieting is not merely whether you do indeed lose weight, but whether, having lost it, you refrain from putting it back on again.**

The approach I have outlined in this book plainly passes that test: at least, it has in my case. As I write, it is now the best part of a year since I got down to my final reduced weight of just under 12 stone, and I have remained at that weight ever since.

I feel better and more vigorous and move and breathe more easily than I did before, and have had an exhaustive health check to satisfy myself that this is not self-delusion. I also no longer experience that rather unpleasant bloated feeling that comes after a particularly heavy meal.

While the business of losing weight required the exercise of a degree of self-restraint and self-denial that was not always easy, particularly at the beginning, I can honestly state that keeping the weight off, once lost, has caused me not the slightest difficulty whatever.

When I was fat, I hardly ever weighed myself. I did not need to be reminded that I was seriously overweight. When I started my diet, as I have already mentioned, I got into the habit of weighing myself every week, to satisfy myself that I was making progress, and to reassure myself that it was worth going through with it. Since reaching my final target weight I have continued the habit of weighing myself every week (indeed there is a temptation, harmless if pointless, to which I occasionally succumb, to do so much more frequently), so as to make sure that my weight remains at that level, and take early corrective action should there be any tendency to edge up or down.

That corrective action can take the form of stricter adherence to the existing regime if your weight shows signs of edging up again, or indulgence in occasional special treats and excesses if it shows signs of edging down. For my part, I have experienced only the occasional tendency for my weight to edge *down* a little, which I have happily corrected in this way.

I do not find it at all surprising that I have experienced no tendency whatever to start putting weight on again, which so many people who have attempted other forms of dieting have complained about. For the essence of the approach set out in this book is the acquisition of a new and sustainable set of eating *habits*; and once your body and mind have become re-educated and re-habituated in this way, it and you will have no wish to change back again. Indeed, I suspect that, in some way, my entire body chemistry has changed to reinforce the habits I originally adopted by an act of will.

### IN THE PUBLIC EYE

What did surprise me was the vast amount of interest my loss of weight and girth aroused when it first became public knowledge. This occurred as a result of a private family occasion at which the *paparazzi* happened to be out in force, and I was among those who had their picture taken. To my astonishment, the next day's papers, broadsheet and tabloid alike, all carried the photograph prominently, alongside one from the old, fat Chancellor days, and marvelled in bold type about the difference.

That was only the beginning. The story, which I had not seen as a story at all, ran and ran. Before long, the columnists and medical correspondents were weighing in (if that is the *mot juste*), and I was inundated with requests from half the newspapers in London to write an article about how I had done it, and from even more television chat shows to appear and tell all. Few of the things I have done in a not uneventful life generated as much media interest as this essentially private and, to be frank, rather banal personal achievement.

Having no desire for personal publicity (even though I had nothing to hide, and speculation that I must be ill could not have been wider of the mark), I turned down each and every request, whether to write in the newspapers or appear on TV. But it did occur to me that if the interest really was as great as it seemed to be, and unsolicited observations from friends and strangers alike suggested that the unexpected media hype did indeed reflect something genuine, then the best thing to do might be to wait and see if the weight really did stay off (which it did) and then write a short book about it.

Hence this appropriately slim volume; which, as I hope I made clear from the start, is not prescriptive but merely descriptive. It tells you what one bona fide card-carrying fattie did to become thin, and how surprisingly easily he did it. But it is not my business to urge you to do the same. If you want to stay fat, then I wish you the best of luck – and suggest you swap this book, forthwith, for a copy of the corpulent Chancellor Helmut Kohl's latest *œuvre, Culinary Travels Through Germany.*

### CONCLUSIONS

I do believe, as it happens, that I am healthier than I was before, although that was not really why I decided to diet in the first place. What I am less sure is altogether healthy is the modern obsession with the shape of one's body, of which the great hoo-ha over 'Lord Lawson's amazing weight loss', to quote one of the tabloids, was perhaps a symptom. Good health has been rightly prized throughout the ages, and it is worth taking a modicum of trouble to keep reasonably fit. But taken to extremes this common-sense desire can lead both to an ugly intolerance towards others, of whom smokers (and I am not one myself) are nowadays the most oppressed victims, and to an absurd self-flagellation, often in what seems like a doomed desire for eternal youth.

The great thing I discovered was that I could lose as much weight as I wanted to lose and still enjoy my food as much as I ever did. Just what that food was, and how it was cooked, is the subject of the second part of this book.

# PART TWO

# Thérèse's Contribution

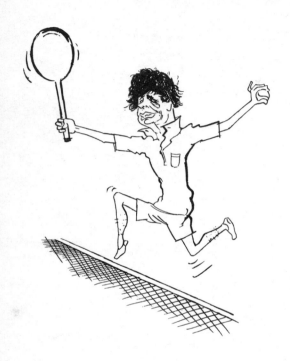

# 4

# Clean Sweep

——

When I first met Nigel, he was forty, feisty and fat. Some way into our relationship, and after many misunderstandings about punctuality, I got the hang of the way Nigel viewed and organized his life, which was in essence based on set meal times, with meetings and life slotted in between. He would describe himself as 'in pain' and 'unable to function' pre-meal.

It was typical of Nigel, when twenty years later he finally decided to lose weight, to be absolute about it and to enunciate the few, simple rules he had concocted. He is good on principles, cutting through the undergrowth. Rising to the practicalities, however, was a challenge: Nigel's ideas of slimming meals like Dover sole and spinach were all very well if being taken out for lunch but hopelessly extravagant in real life and impractical for the rest of the family on a long-term basis.

Not feeling hungry was a prerequisite of Nigel's diet, as was regularity. His brief to me was that he wanted to continue to have three meals a day at the usual times, and that they were to contain nothing on his prohibited list. In practice, this meant low-fat, sugar-free, and low-starch foods, bearing in mind that life cannot be sustained solely on lettuce leaves if it is to have any quality.

I was anxious that our new eating should also be healthy, adaptable for our children and even guests, and not too expensive. The first thing I did was *sort out the larder*: a nasty job unearthing, as it did, embarrassing 1992 date stamps and musty dried herbs, even a burst can of pilchards in tomato sauce. I had to keep a few things that were not on Nigel's approved list, like flours. But I put sugars, maple syrup, marshmallows and the like in a different cupboard for use by others in their coffee or with puddings; and I gave away to a school bazaar tins of sweetened fruit, cake mixes, cooking chocolates. We now have a separate cupboard where the children can find cereals, jams, jellies, crisps, biscuits, hot chocolate and chocolate flakes, and so on.

These procedures decluttered my mind for cooking under the new rules. I myself felt thinner (even though I wasn't) and mentally irrigated. I found it easier to stick to Nigel's criteria when faced in my store only with ingredients that were permissible, in much the same way as a ruthless wardrobe sort-out limits the agony of choice of what top to wear with what bottom every morning. Additionally, once you adopt this approach to cooking – i.e. cooking only with limited ingredients – many problems disappear: jam is really not much use if you haven't got toast. Conversely, toast is less tempting without butter and jam.

The next step was to study the wide range of *reduced-fat products* that are available, and to see which substituted satisfactorily in my recipes. I got a pleasant surprise, in particular with low-fat dairy products. In fact, our family butter consumption has gone down by at least 75 per cent, though on Nigel's maintenance diet, I still use butter (unsalted for preference) when its absence would spoil things, e.g. a small slab for the beginning of a soufflé or any cheese sauce – which, however, can thereafter be made to a high standard with semi-skimmed milk and reduced-fat cheddar cheese.

An advantage of substituting less fattening ingredients in your usual recipes is that it feels less miserable because you are continuing to enjoy many of your favourite flavours and are much less aware of the effort. Going from steak to lentils could be viewed as a radical change and a punishment – only short term, one hopes. But having with fish instead of hollandaise a light lemon sauce (see 'Tricks') of similar flavour is very much less traumatic and is therefore more likely to become a long-term habit. It feels less of a deprivation.

We got to know oils better (and I pondered the significance of polyunsaturates and mono-unsaturates) and discovered some distinct and lovely flavours. You don't want to go mad with oils, though, as they are far from unfattening. And the flavours of interesting leaves were a new discovery too. In his earlier incarnation Nigel despised salads as food for rabbits; now he complains if there isn't a salad available. Salads comprise a vital part of his new eating pattern.

We also revised our attitude to both *proportions and portions*. Used to thinking of meat or fish as the main focus of any dish, vegetables ran the risk of being merely nice appendages. Now we make quite a fuss of our vegetables, enjoying them cooked to perfection (mostly steamed) and discovering that seasoning them after cooking with lemon juice, salt and freshly ground black pepper brings out a fine flavour that seems preferable to that of buttered vegetables. We both like our vegetables so much now that it is easy to eat more, in proportion to the meat or fish, than before, a factor that I am sure was significant in the diet. It also has the virtue of balancing the budget – what we save by eating more vegetables contributes to the cost of quality lean meats and fish.

Nigel soon became more used to lighter foods, to the feeling of being a little less than completely full. I noticed that gradually he reduced his portions and resisted 'just finishing up'. The dog became the beneficiary, but she herself is now having to go on a diet. She and I both got fed up with being asked if she was pregnant.

*Sauces* were rather more difficult to tackle, especially as they are one of Nigel's favourite things. Necessity is the mother of invention. I often now mouli the liquid and vegetables I have slow-cooked the meat or game in, which makes a very acceptable, thick sauce. Flour doesn't come into it, but you can stir in at the last minute some half-fat crème fraîche or low-fat yoghurt if you want a more creamy sauce. Now I make thin but highly flavoured gravies, avoiding thickeners of any kind. And, while a sea bass baked with fennel and lemons *en papillote* tastes wonderful just so, everyday fish has always been enhanced by forbidden sauces such as hollandaise. Instead I make a non-fattening lemon sauce for plain fish or poultry.

Dressings for the salads have developed into an art, choosing from a range of oils to go with the particular ingredients, scattering seeds to add crunch instead of croutons and lardons, and usually using freshly squeezed lemon or lime juice. Though some of the more exotic vinegary dressings on sale can be a delight, I tend to avoid them because many contain sugar.

The key changes to my cooking, then, were:

* incorporating into my recipes all the acceptable substitutes I could think of – not just the obvious low-fat alternatives on sale in the supermarkets, but, for example, using lean pork instead of fatty belly when making a pâté;
* providing meals with more vegetables and correspondingly less meat;
* eliminating the classic sins such as puddings and cakes.

With these changes, which still enable you to cook and enjoy cooking delicious meals, you are already halfway to a permanent, lower-fat and less fattening – and healthier – way of eating, and to becoming and staying slim. If we weren't foodies before (which we both were) we certainly are now. But the term seems to have lost much of its pejorative tone.

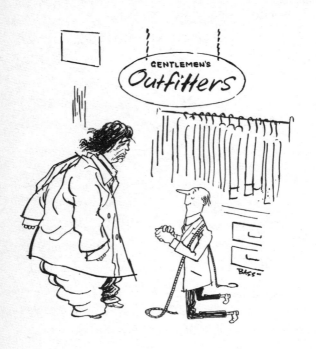

# 5

# Pattern of Eating

———

Nigel has a very different lifestyle these days from when he was in the thick of politics. He has built an office in the disused stables at our home in Northamptonshire, complete with telephone, fax, computer and the like. This means that he can work – and eat – at home very much more than before. Obviously he travels a lot and has meetings in London. When he began his diet in earnest, I encouraged him to select fish as much as possible when eating out, not only for its lightness in dietary terms but because I am not keen on cooking fish all that often at home since its smell pervades the whole house and sets the cats alight.

## BREAKFAST

Nigel makes his own breakfast first thing in the

morning and long before I am conscious. He has
the same every day – poached eggs on toast (I bought
him a two-egg poaching pan) and grapefruit juice.
It takes two minutes to make the juice from two
fruits, either with one of those cheap electric
squeezers or in the manual, compressing one. Very
occasionally, however, we vary breakfast if we are
away or have guests. Equally virtuous cooked breakfasts are kippers, done in the microwave, grilled
or jugged (no butter); or poached or microwaved
smoked haddock with egg on top. Guests sometimes like large platters of peeled and sliced fresh
fruit or unsweetened muesli with proper apple
juice instead of milk.


### LUNCH


When Nigel is working at home and has lunch
here, and if I am in, we have a one-course meal,
followed by citrus fruit when he was reducing,
but on his maintenance diet, a cheese as well, with
a couple of oatcakes or similar (no butter) and
radishes. The things we have for lunch include the
following (asterisked dishes are those which came
on the menu only after he had ended his reducing phase):

A large bowl of **rocket leaves and tinned tuna** (in water, not oil), with pitted black olives, hazelnut oil and lemon juice

----

Masses of filling **celeriac, onion and carrot soup** made with a light stock and moulied – or parsnip, apple and chestnut soup or fresh beetroot soup or a range of many other vegetable soups, depending on what is around

----

A huge bowl of **mussels** (so cheap) poached in dry white wine with shallots, garlic, basil leaves and finely chopped plum tomatoes – it becomes a soup as well as a substantial meal

----

**Parma ham or** *jambon de Bayonne* with melon, figs or papaya, scattered with ginger flakes and black pepper

----

Loads of **mushrooms** (of exotic varieties, when obtainable) steamed in the microwave with a very little olive oil, lemon juice and crushed coriander seeds and served warm

----

**Gazpacho** in summer made from tomatoes, green and red peppers, cucumber, garlic and onions

----

**Asparagus**, when in season, steamed, with lemon juice, salt and pepper added afterwards

———

**Globe artichokes** with lemon and safflower oil dip

———

**Piperade** – made in a few minutes on the top of the stove with eggs and lovely Basque vegetables seared in a little olive oil

———

Poached **smoked haddock** (beware of pre-pared packs which often include butter) on a bed of steamed fresh spinach, with or without a poached egg on top (a light lemon sauce goes well with this and it makes a good supper dish too, especially if you can smarten it by using bantams' or quails' eggs)

———

Left-over **fish soup** – made from salmon bones and bits (after we've had a poached salmon), fish stock, roughly cut vegetables and, finally, an egg and lemon liaison with a few prawns, mussels, and scallops thrown in if available

———

Microwaved **mushrooms and lightly poached scallops** in lemon juice, served *tiède* and peppered, and on dark green leaves; even better with the thick little bacon chunks you

can buy and dry-roast for a few minutes, but
this then becomes *

---

**Omelettes** with mushrooms, tomatoes or
reduced fat cheese (* if cheese)

---

**Carpaccio** with thinly shaved parmesan, a few
drops of olive oil, basil and rocket leaves

---

Mozzarella or feta **cheese salad**,* with tomatoes (preferably of the plum variety), pitted
olives, and fresh basil leaves, served with lots
of pepper and a drizzle or two of olive oil

---

**Cheese soufflé**,* made with the minimum
amount of unsalted butter and flour, but then
with reduced-fat cheddar cheese and semi-
skimmed milk

---

**Pâtés*** of various kinds, made with chicken or
pigs' livers, duck breast (with all fat and skin
discarded after lightly dry-roasting), lean minced
pork (I buy fillet and mince it myself), pheasant
meat (skin off), hare, etc – and using a light
stock and half-fat crème fraîche or fromage frais
instead of cream (see recipe in 'Tricks')

---

Mini **broccoli and cauliflowers**,* or leeks,

steamed, then crisped in the oven with a light cheese sauce (like the soufflé, using reduced-fat products); tinned **palm hearts** done similarly make a change

———

**Celeriac bake**\* – slices of celeriac and finely chopped onion baked in semi-skimmed milk, pepper and nutmeg (like a *dauphinois*)

And endless large bowls of salad. Nigel has a quirky thing about multi-coloured salads. Tomatoes, red peppers and finely chopped red onions are OK together, rocket and spinach ditto. But lettuce and tomato together, no.

I buy all sorts of different salad leaves now – rocket (which I am trying to grow: it is very expensive to buy), sorrel, watercress, young spinach, oak leaf lettuce, lambs' lettuce, flat-leaf parsley, ruby chard, mustard leaves. All are easily purchased at the supermarket – we are fortunate, given that we live in the country, to have a Waitrose only five minutes away and Sainsbury's and Tesco within fairly easy reach. Sometimes the herbs and leaves are sold in growing pots, which add to an earth-mother feeling in the kitchen. (One or two have flourished when I've planted them out in the garden.) One, two or at most three different types of leaves together in a salad seems best as you can really taste each one that way.

Then it's a matter of the dressing and trimmings. Favourite is simply hazelnut oil and freshly squeezed lemon juice. Walnut oil is good too. Occasionally I'll lighten very low-fat yoghurt with lemon juice and wafer-thin slices of crisp apple, easily shaved with a potato peeler, to make a tangy dressing. Lime juice makes a change and I sometimes scatter the salads with judicious portions of crunchy seeds – pumpkin, sunflower, pine kernels, for example. I also cut in fresh herbs from the garden whenever possible – liberal amounts of basil with a tomato salad being the obvious example. Mint is particularly enhancing with grapefruit salad, strips of root vegetables like celeriac, or in a yoghurt dip. Raw fennel is a wonderful salad ingredient. The variations are infinite, given a little imagination.

Depending on your hunger quotient, and sometimes if we want to have a light supper after Nigel has had a business lunch, we will supplement the sort of dish I've just described with a bowl or two of soup – usually made from root or leaf vegetables in a stock, comforting and filling (or refreshing, if a cold soup served in summer). Traditional 'cream' soups can be easily imitated, if that is what you want and in a less fattening way, by swirling in at the last minute, some half-fat crème fraîche or low-fat yoghurt. But consommé-type bases with strips of your chosen ingredients bulking it up, like a Chinese restaurant soup, make a very acceptable first course too.

Or we will have two 'lunch' items, e.g. soufflé and a salad; pâté and salad. And, since Nigel has been on his maintenance diet, he sometimes has cheese afterwards too — Stilton is his favourite, which I buy in a large scoopable round. For a pudding feel, it is delicious with fresh, unsweetened mango chunks which can be bought from the supermarket ready-prepared, a real bonus of a service. Usually, though, Nigel has his Stilton with a couple of oatcakes: there has to be *some* cereal bulk in a healthy diet.

## Puddings

Traditional puddings in our family haven't really featured since Nigel's diet. When reducing, he stuck strictly to two citrus fruits to complete his meals or occasionally other light fruits such as seedless green grapes, Cape gooseberries, lychees, strawberries, raspberries, blueberries — but all unsweetened. A platter of peeled and sliced, colourfully arranged fresh fruit makes a lovely-looking pudding. Bowls of fresh chunks of tropical fruits are always enthusiastically received at dinner parties. More and more people are becoming preoccupied with healthy eating.

As Nigel relaxed his regime, I introduced coulis as an alternative to sugar and cream and as a general livener for fruit platters and puddings. It is extremely simple to make: very lightly poach, and then blend to the right consistency, the berries of choice with just two tablespoons of an appropriate liqueur, cassis being the most useful (a bit of a sin, but not a huge one considering how small an amount each person will consume). Rightly or wrongly, I tell myself that in the cooking process alcohol loses not only its potency but also some of its fattening qualities. I have deliberately not looked for the facts on this matter: suffice to say that Nigel has not got fatter on the occasional coulis.

Now and again on colder days we have a hot fruit pudding. Baked apples or pears, poached in wine or a light syrup, in the oven, are as near as I dare get to overstepping Nigel's strict limits. He will, however, give in for summer pudding, properly made with raspberries, redcurrants and blackcurrants. It is lovely with half-fat crème fraîche. While strictly speaking this is prohibited, you still have to remember that it is a far cry from a *pot au chocolat* in the girth-widening stakes, and he used to be a sucker for all that. So, after the first, absolutely strict patch, life is not wholly denial in Nigel's regime, even when it is time for desserts.

### DINNER

As a general rule, dinner is our main meal and is quite often shared with others, so that some cunning is required in order that children and guests aren't left hungry.

Prime lean meats, poultry, game or fish are usually included, with much emphasis on fresh and delicious vegetables. Indeed, if money were no object, what could be better to slim on than a gingery rack of lamb, trimmed of all fat, a strong gravy, and loads of steamed spinach; or a quickly cooked fillet steak, either plain or served with a soft green peppercorn sauce, and poached mushrooms; or a grilled Dover sole, with just-so runner-beans, and a frothy lemon sauce?

In real life, however, one has to stretch both resources and resourcefulness a bit further. In the first few months of his diet, Nigel was strict about his rules and it was generally easier to serve plain meals, which pleased the children too: they like nothing better than a roast. It was at this early stage that we became vegetable aficionados in a

big way, as there was a practical limit, apart from
any other considerations, to how much meat or
fish it was affordable to eat. The usual fillers like
potatoes, roast parsnips or Yorkshire pudding
were off the reducing list.

Filling up with (mainly green) vegetables provided the answer. We grew to like them best when
steamed, and often enhanced with lemon not
butter, and to indulge in the more unusual and
exotic vegetables nowadays frequently on supermarket shelves. Things like 'patty pan' baby
squashes, steamed sorrel, baked fennel, hot beetroot all added variety. Several times at this stage
Nigel pronounced that he wouldn't after all mind
becoming a vegetarian. (An outcry from other members of the family squashed this idea, however.)

More and more frequently, too, Nigel took
to having as a separate course, usually as a first
course, a large green salad. Undoubtedly that
added bulk and helped adjust his appetite – which
quite plainly changed as he became accustomed to
a different emphasis in the foods we chose, and
in fact to eating less overall. I couldn't say whether
he was conscious of the change or not, but I was,
because I was dealing daily with the quantities and
the leftovers. To complete dinner, when reducing, Nigel had for pudding only citrus or other
light fruits, as I already mentioned, but later he

allowed himself cheeses as well, or even a cheesy
or fishy savoury.

Here are some of his favourite dinners, some
of them exclusively 'maintenance' meals (which,
as before, I have indicated with an asterisk) but
of course including the type of thing he had
during his reducing phase, when flexibility was
not his middle name.

**Chicken or guinea fowl**, plainly roasted in a
hot oven, stuffed with a lemon cut in half, and
spread very lightly with olive oil to crisp. When
reducing, Nigel didn't give himself any skin and
I made a strong thin gravy. We have a large
quantity of the best available green vegetables
in season, usually steamed, and possibly a carrot
or celeriac purée too.

----

**Poussin** – one each. They are often available
reduced but in any case are not very expensive
in our local supermarket. They can be quickly
roasted, more or less as for chicken, and served
with gravy or frothy lemon sauce instead of
hollandaise – or done in a casserole, with (say)
leeks, onions, carrots, a few new potatoes (for
the rest of us) and a good, strong chicken
stock, poached in a slow oven. Add a green
vegetable, e.g. sprouts, to the concoction at the

right time or cook separately. This is a dish that you can easily serve at informal dinners if you split the poussins into halves after cooking but before serving, which takes hardly any time or skill with poultry shears.

———

**Turkey**, a little one, 'French roasted' and invariably succulent done this way, is amazing protein-value for money. Seal the turkey in a very hot oven and then cook with a liberal amount of stock (made from the giblets if you can be bothered). Put in any root vegetables you have that need to be used up, for flavour. Dieters don't have to eat them. Splash the bird with some reasonable red wine while it is very hot, then cover the whole pan with tin foil and cook gently. The stock and vegetables, moulied or blended, make a superb, automatically thickened gravy base.

———

**Partridge** in season are good but I think they need help: like **pheasants**, if plainly roasted they can be a gamble and too dry. As they look so partyish, being a one-bird-per-person dish, I like to do them in a sauce, which means they not only keep warm happily, and safely ready in advance while you have the first course, but are also guaranteed to be tender and moist. Nigel's

favourite way to eat both partridge and pheasant
is my cheaty and adapted version of the classic
*vallée d'Auge* way, which is simply a matter of
cooking the birds slowly in a mixture of celery,
onion, apples and stock (flame them in calvados
at the beginning for added flavour) and then
roughly blending the vegetables and cooking
liquid to make a sauce. If this is for a dinner
party, you can carve and arrange the cooked
birds well in advance (Nigel is very good at
this, being, he says, a surgeon *manqué*), cover
with the sauce and tin foil, and be sure of it
coming up trumps. Chopped fresh parsley at the
last minute adds good colour.

———

A similar, favourite cooking base and sauce for
all birds consists of celery, apple and a few
chestnuts, which you can easily get peeled –
frozen, tinned or in vacuum packs. (These
prepared chestnuts are wonderful too in winter
with sprouts or for soups.) The beauty of this
form of cooking poultry and game birds is that
you need only the smallest amount of oil to
start the birds off over the heat, and no flour
or other starchy thickener of any kind.

———

And if you prefer a creamy sauce, simply stir in
at the end half-fat crème fraîche or even very

low-fat yoghurt. On the same principle, part-
ridges, poached with fresh beetroots, onions and
crushed allspice berries subsequently made into
a sauce, are not only delicious but spectacularly
colourful.

———

**Racks of fat-trimmed lamb**, quickly roasted
*à point* with ginger and drained of all fat afterwards, served with a strongly flavoured *jus*,
make a lovely dinner with vegetables of choice
– spinach steamed with half a lemon seems the
ideal to me.

———

**Steak**. We go for the least fatty and most
tender fillet, only now and then since it is so
expensive. You can almost dry fry the steaks, or
of course use the grill, adding at most a dessert
spoon of safflower or sunflower oil. (I am lazy
about grilling, as the pan is such a pest to wash
up, and the process makes the kitchen smoky.)
Sometimes I crush in the pestle and mortar
some soft green peppercorns and smear them
over the steaks before cooking, and I usually
douse the steaks in a few drops of Lea &
Perrins while they come to room temperature.
If you want to make an *au poivre* sauce,* you
can stir into the pan at the end of cooking and
having removed the steaks, some half-fat crème

fraîche and soft peppercorns and serve a little on each steak.

Occasionally during Nigel's strict phase, I bought a piece of fillet and dry-roasted it whole, slicing it into portions when done, peppered or plain. A crème fraîche sauce* makes this dish a little like a type of Châteaubriand and a plain roasted fillet makes the most lovely Sunday joint. But it is extravagant.

———

More fattening than racks of lamb, but nevertheless not forbidden and less expensive, is a large **leg of lamb**\* cooked French-style (in moisture), something we all love on Sundays. Buy the best quality meat you can afford and, sparingly, spread some redcurrant and/or mint jelly over the joint. Rub the skin with olive oil (for some reason, olive oil works better with lamb than other oils), *sel de Provence*, lazy garlic, chopped ginger and sprigs of rosemary if available. Always put your meat on a rack in the pan so that any fat can drip through to avoid the joint sitting in it. Give it an initial boost in a hot oven and sloosh over it a glass of decent red wine, then cover the pan completely but loosely with foil and continue cooking more slowly. When done, be sure to allow the lamb resting time – which is convenient anyway while you cook the vegetables, which rarely improve if kept warm – as the juices permeate the whole joint when it is out of the oven and definitely improve it. A leg of lamb will feed two hungry families (eight to ten) if carved properly, and non-dieters can enjoy the delicious skin.

————

**Pork**.* We don't have pork often now, even though we all like it. The reason is that the nicest pork incorporates rather a lot of fat. The lean meat alone, while OK, is rather uninspiring. If we have it at all, I'll choose a loin joint which, sprinkled with roughly crushed juniper berries and cooked in its entirety on its rack, is far more tender than separated pork chops and indeed has more flavour too – but it is a strong character who can stop himself gnawing at the gorgeous coating which is, like it or not, sheer fat and skin. You can use pork fillet in recipes with sauces, like a *stroganoff*,* which I now do using a variety of the exotic dried mushrooms you can buy in packets at the supermarket much less expensively than one imagines, finely sliced onions, half-fat crème fraîche as a substitute for soured cream, and crushed green peppercorns.

A homely supper for the family consists of a totally lean **smoked pork loin joint** which the supermarkets sell now in the ham section. You can either bake it or simmer it on the top, which I prefer. Carved thinly, you get more than you think. Early broad beans in their pods, if you are lucky enough to have a source, steamed, are sensational with hot ham and a **parsley sauce**\* – the slimmers' version, which I make with skimmed milk, a teaspoon of butter and less than a dessertspoonful of flour. 'Thicken' with loads of chopped parsley.

———

**Hare**\* is neglected these days, due to squeamishness in my case, so I ask the game dealer to prepare it and the only delicate thing to handle then is the bag of blood, which is necessary for a rich jugged outcome. A whole jointed hare, or just the saddle, marinated for a few hours in wine, a little oil, onion, allspice and lemon peel and then casseroled with winter vegetables, makes a wonderful cold weather dinner, especially if accompanied by aromatic mashed celeriac. To achieve a proper sauce, you do need at the end (and with the blood) some lightly cooked redcurrants, port and arrowroot – even on Nigel's diet, there has to be the odd, minor indiscretion.

**Oxtail\*** is another small sin but well and truly
manageable in the overall eating plan, and it is
one of his real favourites. Cook lots of it slowly
with root vegetables in strong stock and spicy
tomato juice, cheered up with a can of
Guinness and various other bits and pieces. The
key to lessening oxtail stew's sinfulness is to
make it the day before and then take off all the
fat that solidifies on the top when it is cool and
before reheating. Whether it is wise or not to
eat oxtail in particular while the BSE problem is
unresolved is a matter of personal choice.

———

I avoid ready-prepared minced beef, sausages,
and other such products because they probably
contain more fatty meat than you want. But the
butcher will mince anything you ask for. With
lean minced lamb, for example, I make a less-
fattening **moussaka**-type dish, with onions,
garlic, blanched not fried courgette slices and a
few skinned and finely chopped plum tomatoes.
It needs good seasoning – crushed allspice,
Lea & Perrins, some strong stock – and finally
baked in the oven, it almost replaces a
comforting shepherd's pie.

———

You can also stuff and bake a **marrow**, without
the usual rice, but with minced lean lamb (or

beef or pork, come to that), again making a
highly-flavoured vegetable concoction to bind it,
for an unpretentious supper.

———

And if it were just us, once Nigel was on his
maintenance pattern, many cheese-based recipes
came into play, such as a **smoked haddock,
onion and cheese pie**\* nicely crisped on top.

———

I don't bother any more with stir-fries or
curries because they are frankly better at our
local Chinese and Indian restaurants, and you
can pick pretty carefully so as not to break
too many rules. Occasionally, however, but
knowing it must remain that, we have a proper
**risotto**\* which I determined to imitate after an
exquisite experience at the Villa d'Este Hotel
on Lake Como. You do have to allow some
butter for the *arborio* rice base, but after that it
is only spring vegetables (for a *primavera*) or
other virtuous ingredients, and lots of slowly
added warm stock. It is such a treat, and you
don't have to have a large portion.

———

Similarly, Nigel now allows himself to join in
**pasta**\* meals which the children so love.
Usually it is 'Emily's Sauce' that we go for
(named after our fourteen-year-old daughter

because it is her favourite and she has learned to cook it for herself). It is a mixture of skinned plum tomatoes, finely chopped onions, garlic, pesto, spicy tomato juice, a little leftover claret, *tartufi* (mushroom and truffle paste), seasonings, all cooked very lightly and quickly in a little olive oil. Sometimes I add prawns or little salami and bacon chunks. Another favourite sauce is a traditional *ragú* cooked slowly and for much longer with chicken livers and lean minced beef. Or simply pesto and cheese sauce* (using low-fat cheddar or similar and semi-skimmed milk). Parmesan, incidentally, shaved very thinly over the pasta or risotto with a potato peeler, is not forbidden. 'Emily's Sauce' is also a very good way to serve lightly poached scallops or strips of chicken breast, and a number of fish mixtures.

## Vegetables

Unless your attitude is one of sufferance towards them, as an eat-up-for-your-health-and-virtue legacy, vegetables deserve consideration of their own and especially in a reducing diet. Indeed, to classify them in one category is a travesty, and the word 'greengrocer' is nowadays a misnomer. There is a remarkable range of colours, textures and shapes to be marvelled at in a modern vegetable department or in a traditional market on the Continent: shiny, inky aubergines, curly broccoli and cauliflower heads, exotic-looking globe artichokes, voluptuous striped squashes, brightly coloured peppers, crimson and white streaked onions, beetroots, deeply coloured leaves such as spinach, Swiss chard or spring greens, and earthy root vegetables. It follows that the treatment of vegetables cannot be lumped into one category.

Before getting on to methods of cooking, it is worth a reminder that there are many vegetables which, often in combinations with one or two others, are delicious eaten raw – shredded or sliced. Especially in summer, they can be of great use in a diet. They are fat-free and, mainly, non-starchy. Because Nigel gets upset by vibrant colour contrasts, and in any case because it is fun to pick and mix, we sometimes put out separate bowls of each ingredient (and the components of dressings). Effectively, it is like shredded crudités. Almost all raw vegetable salads are enhanced with lemon juice, which also stops root vegetables like celeriac discolouring. Vegetables with strips of certain cold meats or fish – chicken, duck breast, ham, smoked trout, smoked mackerel, smoked salmon, prawns, for example – make a good lunch.

When it comes to cooking green leaf vegetables, the golden rules are to use the minimum of water and to cook for as short a time as possible in order to maximize flavour and to retain both colour and nutrients. Resist as much as you dare, in these days of pesticides, washing vegetables overmuch. Steaming or microwaving are both good methods.

It is, inconveniently enough, a fact that green vegetables served immediately taste better than if kept warm like at school; so, whenever practical, cook them at the last stage – not leaving time for any temptation to let butter melt over them. Again, a little fresh lemon juice squeezed over many green vegetables does them a favour. Nutmeg, scraped off with a kitchen knife, is also a good seasoning, especially with spinach, as is freshly ground pepper to taste. (I have a mixture of black and white peppercorns in my main peppermill both for the look and taste.) As much as possible, I steam our vegetables with coarse sea salt in a three-tiered pan on top of the stove, a method which is economical in terms of both fuel use and washing up. Steaming means that they don't get immersed in water and they come out full of flavour. Most green vegetables need only a few minutes – pull a bit out and taste to judge the moment.

One of Nigel's favourite meals when reducing was a large amount of lightly steamed spinach or other good, dark greens with microwaved fillets of salmon, sole or trout served in the middle, with slimmer's lemon sauce. I deliberately describe it that way round because we made the vegetable as much the main component of the meal as the fish or meat.

Mushrooms too are useful – and delicious – to build a dish around, as they are very light in dieting terms if not cooked in butter or oil (which they absorb far too readily). Lots of them, and there are many varieties to choose from, microwaved with a little salt, citrus pepper and lemon juice, are particularly good with lightly poached scallops.

Vegetables can make a comforting meal on their own especially if, once on the maintenance plan, you have them *au gratin*. Steam them gently first and then put them in layers in a suitable dish and use stock or a half-fat cheese sauce to braise them in the oven. Cauliflower or broccoli cheese with mustard, baked palm hearts (from a tin), celery and fennel all respond well to these methods. And mixtures are good too.

A favourite reducing lunch dish was courgettes sliced lengthways, left standing for a while sprinkled with sea salt and under a paper towel to absorb any bitterness, and baked with skinned, chopped tomatoes and a very little finely chopped onion. The juice from the tomatoes provides enough liquid.

Root vegetables do not need nearly so much preparation as conventional wisdom would have it. Only top and tail carrots, for example. Steamed with coarse sea salt, their flavour is better if unpeeled.

Boil beetroots in their entirety and quickly peel afterwards — the skins come off in a second if you plunge them into cold water. Beetroots in white sauce, using semi-skimmed milk, are lovely. So are young broad bean pods — add chopped parsley and a lot of freshly ground pepper.

Jerusalem artichokes, the knobbly ones, make your heart sink if you assume you have to clean and peel them, with all their little lumps and crevices. Instead, boil them as they come for the minimum time and then put them in the blender with a tub of prepared chicken stock jelly, and you have a most delicious artichoke soup. Stir in, when you are ready to serve, half-fat crème fraîche and chopped parsley or chives. It is worth adding that the peel of vegetables like this is a valuable source of potassium in the diet.

Celeriac is an exception in that you do have to peel and chop it, and it is an effort, but I think it is worth it for its special flavour. You can use it thereafter as a potato substitute or with potatoes, but sliced and baked *dauphinois* with perhaps a little finely chopped onion or puréed it really is particularly good on its own account. Like many other root vegetables, it makes a good base for a soup.

Globe artichokes are perfect slimmers' food, not least because they take so long to eat, leaf by leaf, that there's not a lot of time left for having much else. Dip each piece in a peppered lemon and olive oil mix rather than melted butter.

All in all, a more imaginative and therefore more enjoyable, use of vegetables has definitely been a help with Nigel's loss of weight.

### Fish

There is a bit of a problem here. Nigel loves fish and it is of course an ideal and healthy slimmers' food, assuming it is, not fried or *meunière* – but I don't like cooking it much because of the smell. To overcome this, Nigel chooses fish when he is in a restaurant and, in his life, that is quite frequent. He goes for Dover sole, baked sea bass and other luxuries. At home, I've found the microwave a real bonus for cooking fish in small quantities and fine for the two of us because effectively it steams the food in a sealed unsmelly container,

but it is simply not capacious enough for entertaining quantities.

Microwaved **trout**, for instance, is excellent,
quick, easy and cheap. All you need to add to
the whole but gutted fish is the juice of a lemon
and seasoning. Microwave in a suitable dish
with a lid. There are many other varieties of
fish you can buy filleted which can be cooked
similarly, including salmon, and a range of cold-
water white fishes. They can be jazzed up very
successfully with frothy lemon sauce substituted
for hollandaise. Also good microwaved are
smoked haddock and kippers. But oily fish such
as mackerel are, I think, better baked with cut-
up lemons in a foil parcel in the oven.

———

A whole **salmon**, which if 'farmed' you can
buy for less than a tenner, poached in a fish
kettle with a good *fumet*, is something we often
have when there are guests because a whole
something does look good and you can feed a
decent number this way. I like it best served
lukewarm, with fresh peas cooked with spring
onions, and with lemon sauce or a lot of fresh
mint chopped into a 'sauce' made from very
low-fat yoghurt and lemon juice, or with
spinach and sorrel for a *sauce verte* substitute.

This may be a good moment to state the obvious, that of course one cooks accompaniments – in the case of the salmon, Jersey Royal potatoes perhaps – for those who aren't on a regime. Nigel simply refuses such extras but helps himself to bigger portions of green vegetables instead.

A salmon poached as above and left to cool is an ideal summer party lunch dish to have with salad. And you can make a good soup for the next day if you simmer the bones and bits very slowly in the original *fumet*. When strained, ready to reheat, add plenty of chunks of suitable vegetables – carrots, potatoes, courgettes. At the very end and off the heat, whisk in a mixture of beaten eggs and lemon like *avgolemono*, and you have a smooth and strong fish soup which can be the basis of a light lunch menu.

———

**Salmon kedgeree\*** is a popular informal meal and very useful for large numbers as it keeps warm without a fuss. I cut the amount of rice to a minimum and use delicious wild rice (strictly speaking, not a rice at all), which feels so *al dente* and healthy that I cannot believe it is as starchy as absorbent grains of white rice. The salmon is best microwaved and the eggs are

simply boiled, and I add a little very finely
chopped onion or spring onions. You do not
have to amalgamate the ingredients with butter
and cream – a fish stock works very well
instead.

———

Also well within the rules but sadly not greatly
to Nigel's taste are Mediterranean-style **fish
stews** and soups, made with onions, garlic,
tomatoes, white wine and stock. The variations
on this theme are endless. Another way the
children like to eat prawns and other bite-sized
pieces of fish is in a consommé fondue. Strips
of fillet of beef and chicken are also popular
cooked in this way. Make a few dips to have
with them.

**Grouse\*** is Nigel's absolute favourite. They are
easy to cook and because they are a big treat,
I break a couple of rules so as not to spoil
the ship for a ha'porth of tar. Rub over the
bird a little sweet jelly like redcurrant or
Cumberland, and wrap in unsmoked, rindless
streaky bacon. Roast in a hot oven until done
to the point you like. Eat the *croûtes* cooked
under the birds if you must and serve with a
strong, thin game gravy. Delicious with the
grouse are Brussels sprouts and chestnuts,

puréed celeriac (to soak up the gravy) and spinach, Swiss chard leaves *(blettes)* or spring greens. This is the main course Nigel chooses if we have a celebration meal for his birthday or some such, when he will get out his best claret.

He likes to start with caviar if at all possible (Aunt Jemima's Buckwheat Pancake Mix makes excellent blinis), served with proper sour cream. We might then have summer pudding or a plate of prepared fruits with a coulis. And to end, I make a twice-cooked cheese soufflé in a little cocotte. I do not think you could call this either a reducing or maintenance meal, but what I know is that since Nigel started his new eating regime, we have enjoyed this dinner more than once, and his figure still remains as he wants it to be.

As I conclude this essay on his diet, he is away. The children and I are about to sneak out and get fish and chips . . .

# APPENDIX

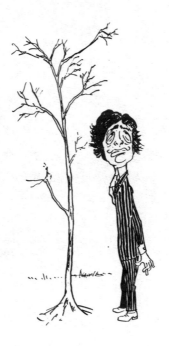

# 'Tricks'

———

A huge help in a diet, and strangely often an effective substitute for butter, **lemons** are indispensable – and not just in tea or with fish. It is scarcely any trouble to squeeze half a lemon on the squeezer as you go along. Use it almost like salt on steamed green vegetables and salad leaves: it highlights flavours and contributes to a liking for seasoned, sharp and pure tastes rather than sweet or muddled flavours. It is the opposite of the sweet-and-sour trend where a glutinous, sugary flavour overwhelms anything underneath, and of the fad for mixing wholly uncoordinated flavours, just to be different.

Lemon juice also enhances some tropical fruits, adds considerably to chicken and other soups as well as to plain poultry dishes, corrects fattiness if squeezed directly over lean lamb chops, and makes a lovely drink: blend cut-up lemons, peel and all, with water and a little honey, then strain.

The zest (not the pith) of lemons and limes, grated or sliced with a potato peeler – use unwaxed fruits – is an asset in **marinades**. Marinating does not necessarily mean lots of oil but a little strong oil like sesame imparts a particular flavour to chicken breasts, say, if combined with the zest and juice of a lime and a splash of soy sauce. Soft green peppercorns rubbed into the surface of a steak or a few drops of Lea & Perrins sprinkled over while you let the meat come slowly to room temperature both flavours and tenderizes. Any meat you plan to casserole, or dark game, benefits from being steeped for quite a time in good red wine, a little oil, and crushed spices of choice. Fish can benefit from marinating for a little while in lemon juice.

✓ **Lemon sauce** is a wonderful dieter's substitute for classic sauces that are yearned for not only because of their shiny texture but also for their lemony tang. Hollandaise is the prime example, but needs far too much butter even to contemplate. Instead, imitate the taste, concept and method as follows:

In a Pyrex jug or pudding bowl, put a little hot (not boiling) chicken or fish stock (6 to 8 fluid ounces) and add the juice of a lemon.

Jellied chicken stock is very good and a fish
stock cube dissolved in the water is quite
acceptable. Whisk in with a balloon whisk
two whole beaten eggs. The sauce will look
opaque and be quite runny – don't be
alarmed. Leave it standing for quite a time
to heat – the simmering oven of the Aga is
perfect but an ordinary oven at a very low
setting (225°F, 120°C, Gas Mark $\frac{1}{3}$ maximum)
will do. Forget the sauce for 45 minutes or
so and then give it a stir with the whisk
again. If it hasn't yet thickened, leave it for a
further half-hour or more. In time, it sets
itself to a thick custard-like consistency and
*voilà*: slimmer's lemon sauce, just as thick,
and nearly as delicious, as hollandaise.

You can also make the sauce in a
microwave if you have a machine with a low
setting. Follow the procedure outlined above
and microwave the sauce for ten-minute
periods until it reaches the right consistency,
whisking inbetween when you check it. All
in all, it probably needs about half an hour
or more.

It is probably best to make this sauce in advance
as it takes so long to set. Then either keep it warm
or, if you made it the day before, you will find that

it reheats satisfactorily in a microwave on a medium setting. (Note: because the eggs are not cooked hard, those who have to worry about salmonella might want to avoid slimmer's lemon sauce.)

Beaten eggs for a **liaison**, whisked in at the end and off the heat, are a very useful enrichening, thickening and smoothing trick, and avoid orthodox starchy thickening or cream. Use them, sometimes with lemon juice, to finalize fish soup for instance, to make it creamy rather than thin and transparent. Or to enrich a cheese sauce (just the yolks).

Less-fattening **cheese sauce** is a standby for all sorts of dishes. Substitute semi-skimmed milk and half-fat cheese for the full cream and full-fat versions and use less butter and flour than normal. It works. This, with egg yolks added at the end, is of course all a soufflé is. Just quickly fold in whisked egg whites immediately before you put it in the oven in a *bain-marie*.

**Yoghurt**, the very low-fat kind, is useful especially in summer as the base for sauces or dips. Lighten even further by whisking in beaten egg white and flavour strongly with chopped fresh mint, basil, cucumber, onion, parsley, sorrel, spinach, or whatever suits. Whisk in a little lemon juice too.

**Stocks and strong thin gravies** have featured in Nigel's diet because plain food frequently benefits from a highly flavoured accompaniment; and, separately, I got used to cooking a number of dishes in liquid, instead of more fattening ways. If pressed, I make no bones, as it were, about using stock cubes or the excellent tubs of jellied stock now readily available. In fact, one of my many cheating fall-backs is a *jus* to serve with meats that is made from a tiny scraping left in the meat pan after pouring off all fat, stirred around with a pinch of flour and a little sweet jelly, to which you add an appropriate stock cube, a little wine, and water if you haven't any proper stock. It works acceptably, and is virtually non-fattening when you consider how little flour each person consumes in the end.

**Poaching, steaming and microwaving** are methods of cooking that have come into their own on Nigel's diet. They all employ only liquid, sometimes even just water, which is clearly a good alternative to methods that require fat or oil. There is an added advantage I observed, which is that as moist-cooked food comes out less dry than the grilled or roasted equivalent, it needs less sauce in general, thus producing a less fattening result overall.

Working on a similar principle, I have found by experimenting that if you get in the habit of **casseroling** many of the usual things much more slowly and for longer, you can frequently avoid the traditional first stage of sealing in hot fat the meat or game component. Make sure you buy the least fatty cuts affordable. Furthermore, you can put a larger quantity of vegetables than you used to in your casseroles, thus cutting down on more fattening ingredients; and make much of the final result, blended, to thicken, avoiding flour, corn-flour and so on.

So-called **'French roasting'** is an effective way of treating joints of meat or poultry using minimum fat or oils, sometimes none. You simply get the meat hot and subsequently cook it in the oven, a little less vigorously than usual, in a liquid that almost steam-cooks. You need a loose covering of foil to achieve this result. However, because the joint becomes very hot to start with, it retains a proper coating and you can crisp it at the end by returning the drained meat to a very hot oven while you deal with the sauce and vegetables.

Anything that produces fat while cooking – a meaty casserole or a stock – benefits by being left to stand until cold, so that you can then **skim off the solid layer of fat** that forms.

Be very careful about **ready-made meals**, including the slimmers' kind which are often less fattening only because they are skimpy in quantity. Ready-made sauces tend to contain thickeners and other processing or preserving ingredients that, apart from sounding horribly chemical, can be unnecessarily fattening.

Serving **sauces and other accompaniments** separately leaves the dieter free to discriminate for himself. For instance, with asparagus I put out both a jug of lemon juice and one with melted butter for everyone to pick and choose, or to mix, for themselves.

Lastly, quite a lot of products are now sold **without sugar** and are a useful aid. Tinned artichokes, tuna in spring water, sweetcorn unadulterated, and fruits with no added syrup are examples.

I have made much of **low-fat versions of dairy products** and they are indeed a real bonus in less-fattening cooking. The best example I can think of is how I cook pâté, which no one thinks of as a diet food and which is filling, cheap, delicious and quite rich. A pâté is very useful in the fridge for Nigel's lunches on his own and, presented in individual scoops or cocottes, a good first course for entertaining. (I like it with a tart apricot coulis.) Slimmers' pâtés are made from livers and lean meats, game or poultry, onions and garlic, spices, a splash of alcohol, eggs and either half-fat crème fraîche or low-fat fromage frais. If you deal with all the ingredients in a food processor before cooking, you can avoid butter or any other fat. I cook my pâtés in a minimal wrapping of bacon, which I then discard, as follows:

*Allow:*

* *around 12 oz (300–400 g) of pigs' and chicken livers, roughly chopped and ½ lb lean pork, chopped or minced*
* *1–2 eggs*
* *up to 1 teaspoon of 'Very Lazy' garlic or fresh, chopped garlic, to taste*
* *salt, pepper and spices*
* *3 tablespoons of stock, preferably jellied*
* *3 tablespoons of alcohol, e.g. white wine or sherry*
* *up to a tub (225 g) of half-fat crème fraîche or light fromage frais*
* *10 slices of thin, rindless, unsmoked streaky bacon.*

Line one or two loaf tins, depending on their size (or a pâté dish or other suitable dish for the oven) with the bacon, stretched as much as possible. Put the tins in a roasting pan to float in warm water (*bain-marie*).

In the food processor, blend all the other ingredients (half at a time if you have only a small machine) leaving aside some of the liquid and fromage frais until you can judge the consistency of the mixture, which should end up slightly elastic and like a thick cream, not too runny. It does not look appetizing at this stage – think of something else, and don't tackle this recipe first thing in the morning. You can blend the mixture coarsely or finely depending on the texture you prefer in a pâté.

Pour the mixture into the lined tin(s) and give it all 15 minutes' boost in a hot oven. Then bake in a slow oven (about 300° F, 150° C, Gas 2–3) for 1½ to 2 hours. (If using an Aga, cook for half an hour in the hot oven, then for up to 3 hours in the simmering oven.)

Pierce the middle of the pâté with a skewer to see if it is cooked. The juices should be clearish and not over-pink, but you don't want the pâté dried out either. Pour off excess juice.

Cool it a bit, invert on to a large plate, and discard the bacon. You can present the

pâté as a whole, decorated with bay leaves
and a few crushed allspice berries, or you
can transfer it to a bowl, or shape it into
egg-shaped dollops (formed with two spoons)
on individual plates and streak a little apricot
coulis around.

This amount is enough for 10 people as a
first course.

You can substitute several other combinations of
choice. For example:

* *2 tubs frozen chicken livers (250 g each) and an
  onion*
* *pack of chopped mixed game from supermarket
  meat departments and 1 tub chicken livers*
* *duck breast, dry-roasted and skinned, and 1 tub
  chicken livers.*

You can also vary the alcohol – Archer's is very
good with a smooth chicken liver pâté, for instance,
if you like it sweetish (use less than you would
wine) and port goes well with a pork pâté – and
the spices: nutmeg is good with chicken livers;
juniper berries (coarsely crushed in a pestle and
mortar) with a rougher pigs' liver pâté.

Pâtés keep very well, if anything improving
after a day or two, and are also fine for freezing.

Lemon Sce. 110.

# Index

———